Mastering Doctor Visits:

Your Guide to Better Healthcare

Charla V. Johnson

BK
ROYSTON
Publishing

BK Royston Publishing
Jeffersonville, IN 47131
http://www.bkroystonpublishing.com
bkroystonpublishing@gmail.com

ISBN-13: 978-1-967282-78-4

Printed in the United States of America

Table of Contents

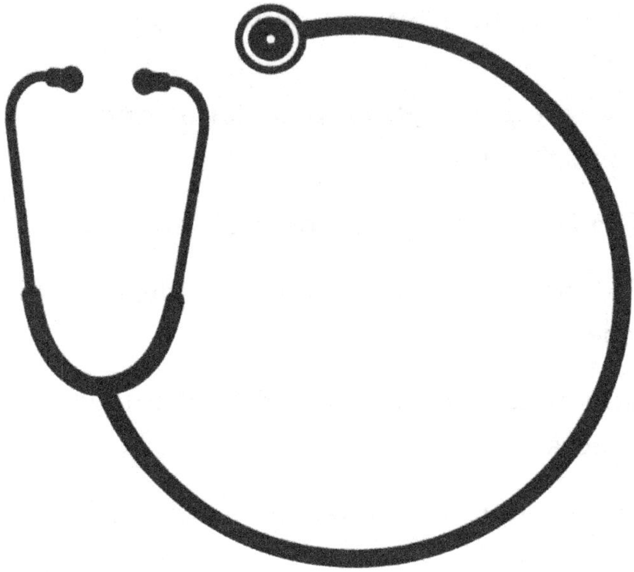

Introduction

This guide is lovingly dedicated to every patient who has ever felt unheard, overlooked, or disempowered within the healthcare system. It is for the individuals who navigate complex medical conditions, juggle multiple appointments, and strive to understand intricate treatment plans, often with limited support. To those who bravely advocate for themselves and their loved ones, even when faced with challenges, this book is for you! It is a testament to the resilience and strength found in seeking and receiving quality care. May this book serve as a companion and a catalyst, empowering you to forge meaningful, collaborative relationships with your healthcare providers and to actively participate in your journey toward wellness. Your voice matters, and your well-being is paramount. This work is offered with my deepest respect for your experience and a fervent hope for a future where every patient feels seen, heard, and valued. It is obvious care changed since the pandemic, but quality and provider compassion should never be altered.

This book also takes into consideration the countless hours that medical professionals have spent to develop and hone skills to provide quality care to patients yet in the present system they are relegated to programs and systems designed to impede the process of care with guidelines which intermittently under mind the knowledge of providers. It is a voice for every frustrated custodian of care who has felt handcuffed by the bureaucracy of the business of healthcare.

The landscape of modern healthcare since the pandemic, while filled with incredible technological advancements and dedicated professionals, can often feel complex and overwhelming for the patient. We enter these spaces seeking not just treatment, but understanding, partnership, and ultimately, a path to better health. Yet, too frequently, the critical element of effective patient-provider communication can become a barrier rather than a bridge. This book was conceived from a deep-seated belief that every individual deserves to feel empowered and equipped to maximize their healthcare interactions. It is born from years of observing the transformative power of well-executed doctor visits—those rare but impactful moments where mutual respect, clear communication, and shared goals lead to tangible improvements in patient outcomes. We aim to demystify the process, providing practical strategies and insightful perspectives to help you transition from a passive observer to an active, informed partner in your own care. Our journey together will explore the foundational elements that foster a productive patient-provider relationship, highlighting the crucial roles both parties play in the matter of communication with your provider. We will delve into the art of preparation for your visit especially with a specialist, the nuances of active listening both for the patient and provider, the power of building trust, and the long-term benefits of consistent adherence to treatment plans.

This is more than just a guide; it's an invitation to redefine your healthcare experience, one appointment at a time, fostering a collaborative spirit that is essential for achieving lasting wellness.

The healthcare encounter is a cornerstone of our well-being, a vital interaction where our health needs are addressed and our bodies' complexities are explored. Yet, the effectiveness of this encounter hinges not solely on the skill of the medical professional, but significantly on the engagement and preparation of the patient. This guide is designed to empower you, the patient, to transform your doctor visits from potentially passive experiences into dynamic, productive partnerships.

We will explore the fundamental principles that underpin a successful patient-provider relationship, beginning with a deep understanding of the context surrounding each appointment. A productive relationship is built on a foundation of mutual respect and clear, open communication, where both patient and provider feel valued and understood. We will outline four critical objectives that should guide every interaction: the imperative of being thoroughly prepared to articulate your symptoms and concerns clearly, the recognition that listening is a bidirectional exchange requiring active participation from both sides, the importance of consciously cultivating a partnership with your healthcare provider, and the commitment to adhering to prescribed treatment plans. We will emphasize the provider's crucial role in initiating dialogue, often beginning with the seemingly simple yet profound question, "How can I help you today?" This opening sets the tone for the entire consultation. Equally vital is our role as patients in actively listening, absorbing the information provided, and asking clarifying questions. The synergy of these actions—clear articulation, attentive listening, and a collaborative spirit—directly influences the quality of care received. Furthermore, we will illuminate how adherence to treatment plans, a direct consequence of positive and trusting interactions with medical staff, is intrinsically linked to improved health outcomes.

Ultimately, this book provides practical advice and encouragement for engaging in collaborative healthcare, underscoring that consistent support and transparent communication are indispensable elements in achieving and maintaining optimal health.

1: Understanding the Healthcare Partnership

The Foundation of Productive Visits

The landscape of healthcare, at its core, is a symbolic partnership. It's a dynamic interplay between individuals seeking to understand and improve their well-being, and the dedicated professionals who possess the knowledge and tools to guide them.

However, it must be understood by the patient that the provider must have the appropriate information about your experience from you. It is paramount that you stay focus on the issues at hand on your visit.

Historically, this relationship might have resembled a benevolent dictatorship, where the physician, as the sole expert, dictated a course of action. The patient, in this model, was often a passive recipient of information and directives, their role primarily to comply. This is often the case in underserved neighborhood, minority or less educated demographics. However, the evolution of medical understanding coming from medical informational platforms such as WebMD, and medical TV spotlights from Sanjay Gupta, MD and Mehmet Oz MD who share medical information in ways that patients have a heightened awareness of health issues. These modalities give patients a growing recognition of unique insights into their own bodies and lives, which has heralded a significant shift in the above model from the matriarchal/patriarchal - patient relation which was initially established. We are moving, thankfully, towards a model of collaborative partnership, where both patient and provider are actively, engaged participants in the journey towards health. A provision of more equity among those with less financial prowess, education, and minorities do not get talked "at", but talked "to" in the medical office now.

This transformation is not merely a semantic change; it represents a fundamental redefinition of roles and responsibilities. A successful doctor's visit, from this modern perspective, is no longer solely measured by the physician's pronouncements or the patient's obedience. Instead, it is characterized by mutual understanding, shared decision-making, and a palpable sense of shared responsibility for achieving optimal health outcomes. It is about fostering an environment where the patient feels empowered to voice their concerns, ask clarifying questions, and contribute meaningfully to the diagnostic and treatment planning process. This active engagement is not just beneficial; it is, in many ways, essential for truly effective healthcare.

The inherent power dynamics within the traditional doctor-patient relationship are undeniable. The physician typically holds a position of authority, built upon years of specialized education and experience. Patients, on the other hand, may arrive at an appointment feeling vulnerable, perhaps experiencing discomfort, anxiety, or a sense of being overwhelmed by medical terminology and procedures. This disparity in knowledge and situational power can, if not consciously addressed, create barriers to open communication and equitable participation. Recognizing these dynamics is the first step for patients to learn how to navigate them effectively. It involves understanding that while the provider's expertise is invaluable, the patient's lived experience of their symptoms, their lifestyle, and their personal values are equally critical pieces of the healthcare puzzle. The provider only has a body part or perceived diagnosis given to them about the patient from an office scheduler or phone operator. The provider has no idea what symptoms the patient is having unless he/she is told by the patient. Oftentimes that information given on the phone is for the schedule may be erroneous.

Fostering a more equitable interaction requires intentional effort from the patient. It is about actively seeking to bridge the perceived gap, not through confrontation, but through preparation, clear communication, and a commitment to engaging as a partner. This does not mean challenging the physician's authority or questioning every piece of advice. Rather, it means approaching the appointment with a mindset of collaboration, where the patient brings their unique knowledge of their health history, their symptoms, their concerns, and their life context – to the table alongside the provider's medical expertise. This shared foundation allows for a more comprehensive understanding of the patient's health status and the development of treatment plans that are not only medically sound but also practical and sustainable for the individual.

Understanding this foundational shift from a directive to a collaborative model is crucial for empowering patients to take a more active role in their health journey. It is also always the skilled provider to actually practice medicine fulfilling their calling to the Hippocratic oath, ..."physician do no harm." It is about moving beyond the passive expectation that a doctor will simply "fix" a problem, and embracing the proactive role of a co-pilot in ones own well-being. This empowerment translates into maximizing the effectiveness of each medical consultation undertaken. When patients are equipped to articulate their needs clearly, ask insightful questions, and participate in decision-making, the potential for accurate diagnosis, effective treatment, and ultimately, better health outcomes, increases dramatically. It transforms the doctor's visit from a potentially intimidating obligation into a valuable opportunity for partnership and progress.

Consider, for a moment, the vast amount of information a healthcare provider must synthesize during any given consultation. They are processing not only the patient's reported symptoms but also their medical history, physical examination findings, and potentially, diagnostic test results. Within this complex web of data, the patient's narrative - their personal experience of their illness - is a vital, irreplaceable thread. When a patient feels comfortable and empowered to share this narrative with detail and clarity, they provide the provider with essential context that might otherwise be missed. This context can illuminate subtle patterns, suggest underlying causes, or highlight factors that might influence treatment effectiveness. For instance, a patient experiencing fatigue might simply report "feeling tired." However, a patient empowered to be a partner might elaborate:

> I feel tired all day, but it's worse after meals, and it's starting to affect my ability to concentrate at work, especially in the afternoons. I've also noticed it's accompanied by a slight dizziness.

This richer description offers the provider significantly more to work with, guiding them towards more targeted questions and investigations. As a patient, you cannot be frustrated with the provider for asking focused questions to gather information because it helps with the differential diagnosis. There are a series of possible causes for your issue, so the questions help us hone in on *your* diagnosis.

The transition to a collaborative partnership also hinges on demystifying the healthcare process. When patients understand the rationale behind tests, treatments, and recommendations, they are more likely to engage actively and adhere to the plan. A provider who takes the time to explain *why* a particular medication is prescribed, *how* it works, and *what* to expect in terms of side effects, is fostering an environment of shared understanding. Conversely, a patient who leaves an appointment feeling confused or uncertain about their care plan may struggle with adherence, not out of defiance, but out of a lack of comprehension or a feeling of being disconnected from the process. The partnership model emphasizes the provider's role in making medical information accessible and the patient's role in seeking clarification and understanding.

Moreover, this collaborative approach recognizes that health is not solely the absence of disease. It encompasses overall well-being, including mental, emotional, and social factors. A patient who feels heard and respected is more likely to feel comfortable discussing these broader aspects of their health. This might include challenges with mental health, difficulties with social support systems, insurance deficits or lifestyle factors that impact their ability to manage their condition. In a partnership model, these elements are seen not as peripheral distractions but as integral components of a holistic approach to care. The provider, in turn, can offer resources and support that address these broader needs, leading to more comprehensive and effective management of the patient's health.

The evolution of the patient-provider relationship also reflects broader societal shifts towards patient-centered care. This philosophy places the individual at the heart of all healthcare decisions and interactions. It acknowledges that patients are experts in their own lives and have the right to make informed choices about their health. The partnership model is the practical manifestation of this philosophy. It's about moving away from a paternalistic approach, where decisions are made *for* the patient, towards a shared-decision-making model, where decisions are made *with* the patient. This requires providers to be skilled communicators, active listeners, and respectful collaborators, and it requires patients to be prepared, articulate, respectful listeners to the trained medical professional, and engaged participants.

The benefits of this shift are profound. When patients feel like active partners in their care, they are more likely to:

Adhere to treatment plans: Understanding the 'why' behind a treatment, and feeling involved in its creation, significantly increases the likelihood of following through with medications, lifestyle changes, and follow-up appointments.

Report symptoms accurately and completely: A trusting relationship encourages patients to be more open and honest about their experiences, leading to better diagnostic accuracy.

Ask clarifying questions: Feeling empowered to seek understanding reduces confusion and potential errors in care. Do not be afraid of what you do not know, you are there with the expert whose job it is to explain things so that you understand.

Experience greater satisfaction with their care: Being heard, respected, and involved fosters a more positive and less stressful healthcare experience.

Achieve better health outcomes: The combination of accurate diagnosis, effective treatment, and active patient engagement naturally leads to improved health results. Patients tend to do better with compliance when they understand how something will help them. Providers need to feel confident that you will comply with the treatment plan. If you are not going to do it before they give you the medication, prescription for physical or speech therapy, just tell them why. If it is financial, transportation, time off work the provider may be able to offer something that will work for your life situation.

Ex: I often want to know the occupation of a person before prescribing blood pressure medication. I do not want to put a construction worker who is outside in the heat on a diuretic when it can easily cause the patient to be dehydrated, dizzy, and or it is difficult to find a restroom.

Ex: Libido is important to the human psychic and should be addressed and considered by the provider when offering medications. Blood pressure medications and some psychiatric medications can suppress this desire and that must be just as important to the provider as it is to the patient. If it is not considered and it affects the patient's life in a negative way, you will lose the confidence of that patient because they feel you do not care about what is important to them.

To truly embrace this foundational shift, patients must cultivate a proactive mindset. This involves viewing each doctor's visit not as a passive event to be endured, but as an active opportunity to gather information, make informed decisions, and contribute to their own well-being. It requires a willingness to prepare, to speak up, and to engage in a dialogue with their healthcare providers. This empowerment is not about challenging the medical establishment, but about becoming an informed and active participant in one's own health narrative. It is the cornerstone upon which all subsequent productive interactions with the healthcare system will be built.

The journey towards a successful healthcare partnership begins long before you step into the examination room. It is a mindset, a preparation, and an active engagement with your own well-being. Understanding that your role has evolved from a passive observer to an active participant is the critical first step in transforming your healthcare experiences. The outdated model, where the physician held all the knowledge and the patient simply followed instructions, is no longer the most effective or empowering approach. Today, the emphasis is on collaboration, on shared decision-making, and on recognizing that the patient's unique insights on their health experiences are as vital as the provider's medical expertise.

This fundamental shift in the patient-provider relationship is a cornerstone of modern healthcare. It acknowledges that health is a complex interplay of biological, psychological, and social factors, and that optimal outcomes are achieved when all these dimensions are considered. The physician's role remains indispensable, providing the scientific knowledge, diagnostic skills, and treatment strategies. The insight that we have on the health industry and business of medicine is paramount for the patient's understanding of what we know and why certain decisions are offered for patient care.

However, the patient's role is equally crucial: bringing their lived experience, their symptoms, their concerns, their values, and their lifestyle into the conversation.

When these two distinct but complementary perspectives converge, a truly powerful partnership is forged.

The inherent power dynamics that have historically characterized the doctor-patient relationship are not to be ignored. Often, patients arrive at appointments feeling vulnerable, perhaps experiencing pain, anxiety, or confusion about their health. This vulnerability, coupled with the provider's position of authority derived from specialized knowledge and experience, can sometimes create a barrier to open communication. However, recognizing these dynamics is the first step in actively reshaping the interaction. It's about understanding that while the provider is the expert in medicine, you are the expert in your own body and your own life. Your experiences, your symptoms, and your understanding of your daily routines are invaluable pieces of information that can significantly inform the diagnostic and treatment process.

To foster a more equitable interaction, patients can adopt several strategies. Preparation is paramount. This involves taking the time before your appointment to organize your thoughts, gather relevant information, and articulate your concerns clearly. Think of it as preparing for an important meeting; the more prepared you are, the more productive the outcome will be. This preparation might include reviewing your medical history, noting down any changes in your health since your last visit, and compiling a list of specific questions you want to ask. By arriving with organized information, which includes a list of your medications with doses. When you are engaged you are not only helping yourself, but you are also demonstrating to your provider that you are a serious participant in your care.

Furthermore, understanding the evolution of the patient-provider relationship empowers you to ask for what you need. If you don't understand a medical term, a diagnosis, or a treatment recommendation, it is your right and your responsibility to ask for clarification. A simple phrase like, "Could you please explain that in a way I can understand?" or "What are the main benefits and risks of this treatment for me?" can open the door to a more thorough explanation and a deeper level of understanding.

This active pursuit of knowledge is not confrontational; it is a fundamental aspect of partnership. It ensures that you are making informed decisions about your health, rather than passively accepting directives.

Ex: I had a seventy-nine-year-old patient that wanted an explanation as to why he had to have an MRI of his brain to examine his hearing nerve for a hearing loss that he had since 2015. It got worse in his right ear in 2022. However, it has been stable for 3 years. The audiologist who ordered it technically was right to order it per protocol, but she never considered the patient's desires. What are his fears for getting an MRI; the age of the patient for the consequences if there was an abnormality found; and the real need for the test at all. We discussed the medical options at length as we reviewed all his audiograms. I asked about his fears of the MRI and radiation; there is none, it is a magnetic field. I talked candidly about his age and health conditions, that if there was a mass lesion they are benign and very slow growing about 1-2 mm annually. He was not having any dizziness, ringing in the ear, or headaches. I let him know that being asymptomatic with three years of stable change in his hearing he could choose to ***not*** get the MRI as long as he understood that I have no way of assessing why his hearing is progressively getting worse. If he agrees with me and him not knowing the status of that area of the brain possibly having a benign growth, he was free not to get the MRI. He should repeat the hearing test in one year. He was happy because his decision was considered. He asked "what would I do?" I told him it is not for me to decide, I have given you all the information that you and your wife need to talk it over and you can call me back with an answer based on an informed decision.

The effectiveness of a doctor's visit is, therefore, significantly enhanced when patients view themselves as active contributors to their healthcare team. This means being honest and forthcoming with information, even if it feels embarrassing or insignificant. Minute details about your lifestyle, your diet, your sleep patterns, your use of alcohol / drugs to include street drugs, or your stress levels can often provide crucial clues for your provider and can prevent the provider from hurting you while trying to help. For example, mentioning that your new medication causes a specific side effect, even if you are not sure it is related, can help your doctor identify a problem that might otherwise go unnoticed. Being truthful about illicit drug use is paramount so providers do not hurt you with treatment plans. **Ex:** I was treating a lady for nosebleeds. I asked if she was using drugs because the inside of the nose had an appearance that a rat had gnaw at the tissue. I kept treating her with antibiotics and using Flonase. I had to send her to the surgeon because I could not get her better. When the surgeon saw me he let me know she confessed to using cocaine daily. Providers are trained to look for and note certain behaviors, and side effects, especially in new medications because those get reported into the companies database and Food and Drug Administration MedWatch site. This open communication builds trust and allows for a more accurate and comprehensive assessment of your health.

Building this foundation for productive visits is a continuous process. It involves cultivating a mindset of collaboration and actively seeking to engage with your healthcare providers. By understanding the shift from a directive to a partnership model, and by employing strategies for preparation and clear communication, you can transform your doctor's appointments from potentially passive experiences into dynamic, empowering opportunities to take control of your health journey. This proactive approach not only maximizes the effectiveness of each consultation but also fosters a deeper, more trusting relationship with your healthcare team, ultimately leading to better health outcomes and a greater sense of well-being. The ultimate goal is to ensure that every visit contributes meaningfully to your overall health and entitles you to live your healthiest life.

This is the essence of the modern healthcare partnership - a shared commitment to your well-being, built on a foundation of mutual understanding and active participation. It is about recognizing that you are not merely a patient receiving care, but a vital partner in the pursuit of your own health. This perspective shift is transformative, enabling you to navigate the healthcare system with greater confidence and achieve more positive and sustainable health outcomes.

Beyond the Waiting Room: Setting the Stage

The journey towards a truly effective healthcare partnership commences not within the confines of the examination room, but well before you even arrive at the clinic. It is a process rooted in thoughtful preparation and a proactive mindset, designed to transform a potentially routine appointment into a powerful collaborative session.

Think of it as preparing for any significant undertaking in your life - whether it's a crucial business meeting, a challenging exam, or an important conversation. The more diligently you prepare, the greater your ability to navigate the situation with clarity, confidence, and a focus on achieving your desired outcomes. In the context of healthcare, this preparation is not merely about convenience; it is fundamental to ensuring that your limited thirty minutes of time with your healthcare provider is maximally productive and contributes meaningfully to your overall well-being.

The initial step in this preparatory phase involves a comprehensive review of your personal health information. This might sound daunting, but it is a manageable process that can yield significant benefits. Begin by gathering any recent medical records, test results, or summaries from previous consultations. Many healthcare systems now offer patient portals that provide easy access to this information, often allowing you to download or print relevant documents. Some major healthcare systems have easy access for you as a patient by contacting medical records online for you as a patient to request sharing of your records with another entity. In case you did not know the HIPPA laws protect your personal medical information, you are the only one that can request your medical records be transferred to others. HIPPA stands for Health Insurance Portability and Accountability Act of 1996. If you have a primary care physician who coordinates your care, ensure you have a clear understanding of your medical history as they perceive it. This includes a chronological overview of significant diagnoses, past procedures, hospitalizations, and any chronic conditions you manage. Familiarizing yourself with this information allows you to identify any discrepancies or gaps that might need clarification during your appointment. For instance, you might discover that a diagnosis has been recorded incorrectly, or that a vital piece of your medical history has been overlooked. Having this readily available allows you to address these points directly, ensuring accuracy and completeness in your medical profile.

A critical component of your pre-appointment preparation is the meticulous compilation of your current medication list. I recommend that you have a 3 x 5 card with any known allergies along with all the names of your medications, dosage, how often you take them, and what they are for. You should keep this in your wallet or purse at all times. In this day and time, you would think why write it out when you can put it in your phone. However, if you are to fall out in Walmart no one can open your phone. If there were ever a medical emergency and you could not communicate, or a family member or friend is not with you, medical personnel could find this information very helpful for treating you. This is an area where even minor oversights can have significant implications. Your list should also include over-the-counter drugs, vitamins, herbal supplements, and any homeopathic remedies you might be taking. For each item, aim to record the full name of the medication, the dosage (e.g., milligrams, units), the frequency with which you take it (e.g., once daily, twice a day), and the reason for taking it. It is also essential to note any recent changes to your medication regimen. This could include starting a new medication, stopping one, or adjusting the dosage of an existing one. Even seemingly innocuous changes, such as switching from one brand of a common pain reliever to another, can be relevant. For example, if you have recently started taking a new supplement that you believe might be interacting with your prescribed blood thinner, or if you have stopped taking a medication due to side effects, this detail is crucial for your provider to know. Having this comprehensive and up-to-date list readily available allows your physician to assess potential drug interactions, evaluate the effectiveness of your current treatments, and make informed decisions about any necessary adjustments. Many patients find it helpful to create a digital document on a smart phone (however the 3 x 5 card in the wallet is easily assessable to people trying to help you in an emergency as discussed earlier); or a dedicated notebook for this purpose, updating it as soon as any changes occur, rather than relying on memory.

Beyond medications, it's vital to document any significant changes or new developments in your health since your last visit. This requires a period of honest self-reflection. Think about how you have been feeling generally. Have you experienced any new or worsening symptoms? These could be physical, such as pain, fatigue, changes in appetite or sleep patterns, digestive issues, or new skin conditions. They can also be mental or emotional, such as persistent low mood, increased anxiety, difficulty concentrating, or changes in your energy levels or sleep patterns. Be specific in your descriptions. Instead of simply stating "I feel tired," try to elaborate: "I've been experiencing a persistent fatigue that worsens in the afternoon, making it difficult to concentrate on work tasks. This has been ongoing for about three weeks." Similarly, if you are experiencing pain, try to describe its location, intensity, duration, and what, if anything, makes it better or worse. This detailed symptom of reporting provides your provider with valuable clinical information that can guide the diagnostic process.

It is equally important to note down any specific concerns or questions you wish to discuss with your healthcare provider. Often, during the course of a day or week, you might have a thought or a question about your health that you intend to remember, only to have it slip your mind by the time of your appointment. Creating a dedicated list for these queries ensures that each concern is addressed. This list can be quite diverse. It might include questions about a particular test result, a request for a referral to a specialist, a desire to discuss lifestyle modifications, or a query about preventive care measures. For example, you might want to ask about the recommended frequency of a particular screening test based on your age and risk factors, or you might be curious about the benefits of a new exercise regimen you have started. Bringing a list of these questions demonstrates your engagement and commitment to actively managing your health. It also helps to manage the limited time available during an appointment, ensuring that the most important issues are prioritized and discussed thoroughly. It is important for me to mention here that most healthcare systems promote some type of digital communication with your provider. If you have that type of access to your physician, utilize it to send your questions and concerns.

When you are with a specialist focus on the body system you are being seen for. An example if you are seeing the cardiologist for your heart palpitations and skipped beats, discussing your sinus pressure or discussing abdominal pain or loose stools with him is not useful information to the cardiologist.

Furthermore, preparing for your appointment involves considering the practical aspects of your visit. If you are seeing a new provider or visiting a new clinic, take a moment to locate the facility beforehand, understand parking arrangements, and note the clinic's operating hours. Knowing how to get there and what to expect upon arrival can significantly reduce pre-appointment anxiety. If your appointment requires fasting, ensure you adhere to those instructions meticulously. If you need to bring specific documents, such as insurance information or a list of your medications, have them readily accessible in a designated folder or bag. Being physically and logistically prepared allows you to focus your mental energy on the health-related discussions during the appointment itself.

The mental preparation for a doctor's visit is just as crucial as the physical and informational aspects. This involves cultivating a mindset of open communication and a willingness to be an active participant. Recognize that your provider is there to help you, and that sharing information openly and honestly is essential for them to do their job effectively. Approach the appointment with a collaborative spirit, understanding that you are entering into a partnership. This means being prepared to answer questions truthfully, even about sensitive topics such as diet, exercise, alcohol consumption, substances such as illicit drugs or vaping or sexual health. Remember that healthcare professionals are accustomed to discussing these matters and their sole aim is to understand your health context better. Providers are not there to judge behavior but to help facilitate what is best to maintain an optimal quality of life for you as the patient. If you feel hesitant or embarrassed, remind yourself that the information you provide is confidential and will be used solely for the purpose of improving your health. The only thing not confidential that you divulge to your physician is if you have committed a crime such as rape, incest, or murder.

Another aspect of mental preparation is to manage your expectations. While you are an active partner, your healthcare provider remains the expert in medical diagnosis and treatment. Understand that they may not have all the answers immediately, and that further tests or consultations might be necessary. Be open to their recommendations and be prepared to discuss different treatment options, weighing the pros and cons together. If you have specific preferences or values that might influence your treatment decisions, such as a desire to avoid certain medications, religious preferences or cultural beliefs, or a preference for non-invasive therapies, it is important to communicate these clearly and respectfully. This allows for shared decision-making that aligns with your personal beliefs, along with incorporating important medical scientific information that your provider can share to enhance your quality of life.

Consider the environment of the waiting room as an extension of your preparation. While waiting, resist the urge to immerse yourself solely in your phone. Instead, use this time to mentally review your prepared notes, your list of questions, and your medication details. This quiet period can also be an opportunity to center yourself and focus on the purpose of your visit. If you are feeling anxious, simple deep breathing exercises can be very effective in calming your nerves. The goal is to arrive at the examination room feeling composed and ready to engage, rather than rushed or overwhelmed.

In essence, preparing for a doctor's appointment is about taking control of your healthcare journey. It transforms you from a passive recipient of care into an informed, engaged, and active participant. By dedicating time to review your health records, meticulously list your medications, document your symptoms and concerns, and prepare yourself mentally and logistically, you are setting the stage for a more productive, insightful, and ultimately, more effective healthcare experience. This proactive approach is not just about optimizing the immediate interaction; it is about building a strong foundation for a lasting and trusting partnership with your healthcare provider. This is crucial for achieving and maintaining optimal health in the long term. Each step taken in preparation is an investment in your own well-being. This ensures that when you finally sit down with your doctor, you are both equipped to work together seamlessly towards your health goals. This diligence in preparation is what truly elevates a standard medical visit into a powerful collaborative effort.

The initial moments of a healthcare encounter often

sets the tone for the entire consultation, and the provider's opening question, "How can I help you today?", is far more than a simple pleasantry. It serves as a foundational invitation, a deliberate gateway into the dialogue that will shape the course of your care. This seemingly straightforward question is the provider's primary tool for understanding your immediate needs and priorities. For the patient, however, it represents a critical opportunity - a chance to steer the conversation from the outset, ensuring that the most pressing health concerns are brought to the forefront.

Think of this opening as a well-crafted prompt for an essay. The quality of the response, the clarity of the ideas presented, and the logical flow of information will directly impact the overall success.

Similarly, how you respond to "How can I help you today?" can profoundly influence the effectiveness of your doctor's visit. It's not about simply listing every minor ailment you might be experiencing; it's about identifying and articulating the core reason for your visit, the issue that is most significant to you at this moment. I have had patients tell me; "well, I have had this issue for 15 or 20 years." To the provider the next series of questions are what has been done for this in the past; and if nothing has been done or you never mentioned it before; what and when did it change to make you get help for it now? This requires a degree of self-awareness and the ability to prioritize, skills that are honed through the preparation discussed in the previous sections.

When faced with these questions, the impulse might be to offer a vague or overly generalized response. Phrases like "I'm not feeling well" or "I just need a check-up" can be a starting point, but they lack the specificity needed for a truly productive interaction. Healthcare providers are trained to elicit more detailed information, but by offering a more precise answer upfront, you streamline the process and help them focus their expertise. That is what activates the computer in the provider's brain spoken of earlier in the providers brain that takes your data and inputs it to come up with a differential diagnosis. Consider what brought you to the clinic on this particular day. Is it a new symptom that is causing concern? A worsening of a chronic condition? A need to discuss test results or a treatment plan. Pinpointing the primary driver for your visit is the key to an effective response.

For instance, if you have been experiencing persistent headaches that are interfering with your daily life. A more effective response than "I have a headache" might be, "I've been having severe headaches that occur daily, particularly in the afternoon, and they're making it difficult to concentrate at work. I'm concerned about what might be causing them." This level of detail – the nature of the symptom, its frequency and timing, its impact on your life, and your underlying concern – provides the provider with immediate, actionable information. It allows them to begin formulating hypotheses and planning an appropriate course of investigation.

If your visit is for a follow-up on a known condition, be equally specific. Instead of "I'm here for my diabetes check-up," you might say, "I'm here for my quarterly diabetes review. My blood sugar readings have been a bit higher than usual over the past month, and I'm also experiencing some new tingling in my feet." Again, this provides context and highlights specific areas of concern that require the provider's attention. It signals that you are actively monitoring your health and are prepared to discuss specific aspects of your condition.

It's also important to recognize that "How can I help you today?" is an open-ended question designed to elicit information. It's not an interrogation, but an invitation to share. Resist the urge to feel rushed or pressured into a quick answer. Take a moment, breathe, and access the notes you have prepared. Your meticulously compiled list of symptoms, concerns, and questions is your greatest asset at this moment. Select the most significant item from that list to lead with.

Consider the scenario where you have multiple issues to discuss. While it's tempting to list them all at once, it can be overwhelming for both you and the provider. The opening question is your opportunity to present your top priority. Once that primary concern is acknowledged and addressed, you can then transition to secondary issues. For example, you might start with, "The main reason I'm here today is because I've developed a persistent cough that hasn't gone away in three weeks." After the provider has engaged with this primary concern, you can then add, "I also wanted to mention that I've noticed some swelling in my ankles recently, and I'm due for my cholesterol test."

This structured approach ensures that your most urgent need is met first, while still allowing for a comprehensive discussion of other health matters. As stated above the provider in order not to be overwhelmed and miss something will need to do a focused exam for that key problem.

A cough that has been persistent would seem like a lung issue, but it is important to add in the swelling of the ankles because this may be a cardiac or heart issues that will need all the attention of the provider to rule out congestive heart failure.

Listening to the lungs and heart, feeling the belly for softness and distension, check the legs for pulses and pitting edema is vital so the appropriate tests are ordered. This is not the time to bring up the arthritis from the knee that is bothering you for several years.

The way you frame your response also matters. A tone of curiosity and collaboration is more effective than one of demand or complaint. Even if you are experiencing significant discomfort or frustration, articulating your concerns in a measured and informative way will foster a more positive and productive provider interaction. Instead of saying, "This pain is unbearable, and you need to fix it," or "no one has done anything for me about this", try a more descriptive approach: "I'm experiencing significant pain in my lower back, which is limiting my ability to move. I'm hoping we can explore what might be causing it and what treatment options are available." Simply demanding a particular test or medications is also not helpful to providers. For example, you may desire and MRI for your sinus facial pain because your friend, who is non-medical, told you they had one. However, but that is not the appropriate test for you a CT scan looks at the sinuses and nasal endoscopy (nose camera) would assess you far better than the MRI and would be less expensive for you. Providers know the appropriate test to order and when for the insurance companies to pay for them otherwise you could end up with an astronomically outstanding bill.

> **Ex:** I tried to explain to a patient this very issue. A CT scan is not used for the evaluation and surgery. She insisted on getting an MRI though I explained to her that it would likely not be covered because it is not used as standard care for the sinuses. After a few weeks the test was

completed. As I stated the patient obtained the MRI, but the insurance refused coverage. This cost her $1900 and she still had to get the CT scan later for further treatment for another $800. Because she refused to listen, there was a $1900 overpayment.

Furthermore, the provider's opening question is an invitation to engage in active listening, which is a two-way street. While you are articulating your concerns, pay attention to the provider's body language and verbal cues. Are they nodding, making eye contact, or asking clarifying questions? These are all indicators that they are listening and processing the information you are providing. Conversely, if they seem distracted or dismissive, it might be a signal to rephrase your concern or ask if they have understood correctly.

The effectiveness of your response to "How can I help you today?" is deeply intertwined with the concept of shared decision-making. When you clearly articulate your primary concern, you are empowering the provider to involve you in the process of finding a solution. Trying to impress providers with a diagnosis you have Googled or looked up on WedMD is not helpful in the charge for the provider's computer to be activated for hypothesis of diagnosis. This often clouds the providers judgement for diagnosis and treatment. The provider needs symptomatic information, time frames, previous treatments, and body locations. They can then present options, explain the rationale behind different diagnostic tests or treatment approaches, and engage you in a discussion about what aligns best with your personal circumstances, values, and preferences. This collaborative approach, initiated by a clear and concise response to the opening question, is the cornerstone of a strong patient-provider partnership.

I must say post pandemic office visits have changed drastically from the initial office visit model which was matriarchal/patriarchal patient and collaborative patient - provider model where the patient passively accepts the diagnosis. During the time of the pandemic, office visits were limited with little to no tactile examinations whether office visits or virtual. The patient was to give a short history and most times a recommendation of what they suspected they had with a treatment plan which was largely obtained from one of the medical internet platforms aforementioned. Providers capitulated and the patients would either get better or worse from the guess work without a proper examination. Healthcare was relegated to this model for the 2-3 years during the pandemic. We have now succumbed to a more compromising version of patient provider participation.

It's also worth considering the unspoken expectations embedded within the original question of "how can I help you?" The provider is signaling their readiness to dedicate their time and expertise to your health needs. They are opening the door for you to express what is most important to you. This mutual understanding forms the basis of trust, which is essential for any effective partnership. By taking the time to prepare your response and delivering it clearly, you demonstrate respect for the provider's time and expertise, while also asserting your own agency in managing your health.

For patients who may have communication challenges, whether due to language barriers, hearing impairments, or cognitive difficulties, preparation becomes even more critical. Having a family member or trusted friend present to assist in articulating concerns can be invaluable. Alternatively, utilizing visual aids, written notes, or translation services can bridge communication gaps and ensure that the core message is conveyed effectively. The fundamental principle remains the same: to provide clear, concise information that guides the provider toward understanding and addressing your most pressing health needs.

In situations where you have a complex medical history or multiple chronic conditions, it can be challenging to decide what to prioritize. In such cases, referring back to your prepared list and considering which issue is causing the most distress or has the most significant impact on your quality of life is a useful strategy. You might also consider what specific outcomes you are hoping for from this particular visit. Are you seeking a diagnosis, a prescription refill, a referral, or simply reassurance?

Knowing your desired outcome can help you frame your initial statement. Also, once issues are shared with the provider, it is paramount that you trust them on which is most pertinent to your health and safety to address right away.

The providers themselves often use this opening as a subtle test of how engaged the patient is with their own health. A patient who can articulate their concerns clearly and concisely often demonstrates a higher level of engagement and preparedness.

This, in turn, can influence the provider's approach, leading to a more thorough and collaborative discussion. Conversely, a vague response might prompt the provider to spend more time probing for information, which can consume valuable appointment time that could otherwise be dedicated to problem-solving.

Consider the impact of technology on this initial interaction. Patient portals and electronic health records have made it easier for providers to access a patient's history. However, this digital information is not a substitute for the patient's lived experience and current concerns. Even today not all healthcare electronic medical records systems are linked to share valuable data. This is especially true from state to state and sometimes hospital system to hospital system. Still, the opening question remains the essential human bridge, connecting the objective medical data with the subjective reality of the patient's health. Your ability to articulate your present concerns verbally, even with the support of digital records, is paramount.

Let's delve into specific examples to further illustrate effective responses.

Scenario 1: New Symptom

Less Effective: "I'm not feeling right."

More Effective: "I've developed a rash on my arms over the past week. It's itchy and sometimes burns, and I'm worried it might be an allergic reaction."

Why it is better: This response specifies the symptom (rash), its location (arms), its characteristics (itchy, burning), its duration (past week), and the patient's concern (allergic reaction). This gives the provider a clear starting point for diagnosis.

Scenario 2: Worsening Chronic Condition Less

Effective: "My arthritis is acting up."

More Effective: "My arthritis in my knees has been significantly worse over the last two weeks. The pain is more constant, and I'm having trouble walking upstairs, even with my usual medication."

Why it is better: This response identifies the condition (arthritis), its location (knees), the change (significantly worse), the timeframe (last two weeks), the impact (trouble walking upstairs), and the context of existing treatment (even with usual medication). This alerts the provider to a potential need to adjust treatment.

Scenario 3: Medication-Related Concern

Less Effective: "My blood pressure pills don't seem to be working."

More Effective: "I'm here to discuss my blood pressure medication. My home readings have been consistently in the range of 150/95 for the past month, which is higher than usual, and I've also been experiencing some dizziness."

Why it is better: This response specifies the medication class (blood pressure), provides objective data (home readings), quantifies the change (150/95, higher than usual), gives a timeframe (past month), and reports a related symptom (dizziness).
This is crucial for assessing medication efficacy and potential side effects.

Scenario 4: Routine Check-up with Specific Question

Less Effective: "I'm here for my annual physical."

More Effective: "I'm here for my annual physical. Everything feels generally okay, but I wanted to ask about the recommended screening tests for someone my age with a family history of [specific condition], and also discuss a new mole I've noticed on my back."

Why it is better: This response clearly states the purpose of the visit (annual physical) but also proactively introduces specific topics of discussion that are important to the patient (screening tests, family history, new mole). This shows initiative and ensures these important points are not overlooked.

The provider's question, "How can I help you today?", is a powerful tool for fostering a partnership. It is an invitation to engage, to share, and to collaborate. By preparing your response, identifying your primary concern, and articulating it clearly and concisely, you are not only optimizing your time with the healthcare provider but also actively participating in your own care. This initial exchange lays the groundwork for a more productive, effective, and ultimately, more empowering healthcare experience. It transforms the encounter from a passive receipt of services into an active dialogue, where your voice and your concerns are heard and addressed from the very beginning. This is the essence of building a strong and effective patient-provider partnership, one clear statement at a time.

The journey towards a truly collaborative healthcare experience begins long before you set foot in the examination room. It starts with a fundamental internal process: defining what you hope to achieve during your interaction with a healthcare professional. This act of setting clear objectives transforms your visit from a potentially passive reception of care into an active pursuit of your health and well-being. It is about taking the reins, identifying your priorities, and ensuring that your time with your provider is maximally beneficial. Without a well-defined purpose, even the most skilled and attentive healthcare provider may struggle to address your most pressing needs effectively, simply because they are unaware of what those needs truly are. What is said in this last sentence is vital, we want to help but you have to share a cohesive focused problem with us and *not* proposed diagnosis mixed with multiple symptoms and multiple problems.

Scenario 1: New Specialty Visit

Less Effective: "I've been feeling bad for a minute, doc. My told me to take some over the counter spray stuff, I did once."

More Effective: "I've been having colored mucus, headaches with pressure between my eyes, top teeth hurt, and nasal congestion for the past month. I have called my regular doctor, but I have just used the nasal spray he said a couple of time. It didn't help."

Why it is better: This response specifies the symptom (colored mucus), its location (head, nose), its characteristics (pressure, congestion), its duration (past month), and what has been tried (nasal spray -although not used long enough). This gives the provider a clear starting point for diagnosis and for developing a treatment plan and whether or not to engage other testing. Also, an important note here using slang terms like "it's been a minute" is not realistic at all.

I have said to patients who use that type of jargon in the office. You mean to tell me you woke up, called into work and made an appointment. Got dressed and drove across town to seek my help for a problem you have had for sixty seconds. Their reply is well doc, you know what I mean. I express to them that the English language gives us a definition for a minute being seconds long. I hear people say that to me and for some that means a week to a month, others two months to six months, so, no I do not know what you mean. Timelines for providers mean something and assist us with treatment plans to include when certain images should be ordered. Insurance companies will deny a claim if you have a diagnosis and have not tried any recommended treatment plans to elevate the problem.

Consider the analogy of embarking on a journey. If you set out without a destination in mind, you might wander aimlessly, perhaps stumbling upon something interesting, but unlikely to reach a place that truly serves your original intent. Similarly, a healthcare visit without defined objectives can lead to a meandering conversation, potentially touching upon many aspects of your health but failing to address the core reasons for your concern or the specific outcomes you desire. Your health objectives act as your compass and map, guiding the conversation and ensuring that the encounter remains focused and productive.

My mom used to say the phrase "jack of all trades, but a master of none." What she meant was doing or knowing a lot of things but not mastering or being great at any of them. If your focus is on one or two similar entities better productivity will materialize. I can examine and ask pertinent question to help with the throat pain and food feeling like it is sticking in the chest when you swallow. However, if you throw in a symptom of by the way my ankle has been hurting when I stand a lot also. The series of questions for the ankle pain does not coincide with the problems that the Ear Nose and Throat doctor specializes in. You must keep in mind the mind of the provider is analogous to a computer where data is input, and it hits an algorithm which matches symptoms with appropriate exams, test, medications, and imaging studies to produce a diagnosis.

The process of defining these objectives involves

introspection and a degree of self-assessment. It requires you to honestly evaluate your current health status, identify any changes or concerns, and consider what constitutes a successful outcome for that particular visit. These objectives can range widely, from addressing an acute symptom that is causing distress, to managing the complexities of a chronic condition, to seeking clarification on a newly prescribed medication or treatment plan. They can also extend to preventive care, such as discussing age-appropriate screenings or lifestyle modifications aimed at long-term health. The key is to translate your overall health aspirations into concrete, actionable goals for each specific encounter.

One of the most common and crucial objectives for many patients is managing chronic conditions. These are often long-term health issues that require ongoing attention and management. For individuals living with conditions like diabetes, hypertension, arthritis, or asthma, each doctor's visit is an opportunity to assess the current state, review the treatment plan, and potentially make adjustments. When approaching a visit for a chronic condition, your objectives might include: understanding recent blood sugar readings and their implications; discussing any new pain or mobility issues related to arthritis; evaluating the effectiveness and potential side effects of medication for hypertension; or assessing how well asthma symptoms are controlled and whether inhaler technique is optimal. It's not enough to simply say, "My diabetes is okay." A more defined objective would be, "I want to understand why my HbA1c levels have been creeping up over the last six months and discuss strategies to bring them back into the target range." This provides the provider with a clear focus for the consultation.

Another significant objective for many is the investigation of new or concerning symptoms. When a new health issue arises, it can be a source of anxiety and uncertainty. Your primary objective in such a scenario is often to obtain a diagnosis and a plan for management. This involves clearly articulating the symptoms you are experiencing, their onset, duration, frequency, severity, and any factors that seem to exacerbate or alleviate them. For example, if you've developed persistent fatigue, your objective might be to understand potential causes and identify diagnostic tests that could shed light on the issue.

A well-defined objective here would be: "I want to discuss my persistent fatigue, which has been present for the past month. I'm concerned about potential underlying causes like anemia or thyroid issues, and I'd like to understand what tests can help us investigate this." This allows the provider to systematically approach the diagnostic process.

Understanding and adhering to treatment plans is another vital area where setting objectives can be highly beneficial. Healthcare providers often prescribe medications, recommend therapies, or suggest lifestyle changes. Patients may have questions about how a medication works, its potential side effects, its interactions with other drugs they are taking, or the correct dosage and timing. Similarly, a new physical therapy regimen or dietary recommendation might require clarification on proper technique or implementation. For instance, after a diagnosis and a proposed treatment plan for a new condition, your objective for the follow-up visit could be: "I want to ensure I fully understand the prescribed medication, including its purpose, dosage, potential side effects, and how it fits into my overall treatment. I also want to clarify the recommended exercises for my physical therapy and confirm I'm doing them correctly." This proactive approach ensures that you leave the appointment with the knowledge and confidence needed to follow through with your treatment.

Beyond specific symptoms or conditions, many visits are for routine check-ups or preventive care. Even in these instances, having defined objectives is important.

These objectives might revolve around screening tests, vaccinations, or discussions about maintaining good health. For example, you might want to discuss the appropriate cancer screening schedule for your age and risk factors, or you might wish to inquire about a new vaccination that has become available. A clear objective for a routine visit could be: "I'm here for my annual physical. I'd like to discuss my cholesterol levels from last year, review any recommended vaccinations for my age group, and talk about strategies for increasing my daily physical activity." This ensures that routine visits are not just perfunctory but also serve as opportunities for proactive health management.

Prioritizing your concerns is a critical step in

defining your objectives. It's rare that a single visit can address every single health-related thought or worry you might have. Most people have a running list of minor ailments or questions. When you are in the provider's office, it's essential to identify the most significant issue for that particular appointment. This requires a realistic assessment of what can be reasonably accomplished in the allotted time and what requires the most immediate attention. Ask yourself: What is causing me the most distress right now? What is having the biggest impact on my daily life or my long-term health? What is the most urgent matter that needs to be addressed?

Consider a patient who has been experiencing occasional headaches for a few weeks, has a persistent cough that is bothering them, and is due for a refill of their blood pressure medication. While all these are valid health concerns, they likely cannot all be thoroughly addressed in a single, standard appointment. The patient needs to prioritize. If the headaches are becoming more severe and frequent, that might be the primary objective. If the cough is affecting their sleep or causing significant discomfort, that could be the priority. Or, if there's a concern about the blood pressure medication efficacy or side effects, that may take precedence. The patient might choose to focus on the headaches for this visit, with the objective of exploring potential causes and relief strategies, and then schedule a separate appointment or address the other issues during a future visit. This prioritization ensures that the most critical concern receives adequate attention.

Effectively communicating your objectives to your healthcare provider is just as important as defining them. Once you've identified your goals for the visit, you need to articulate them clearly and concisely, ideally early in the encounter. As discussed previously, the provider's opening question, "How can I help you today?", is your primary opportunity to set the agenda. Instead of a vague statement, you can state your main objective directly. For example, "I'm here today because I'm concerned about a new mole I've found on my arm, and I'd like you to examine it." Or, "My primary goal for this visit is to discuss my recent blood test results and understand what they mean for my ongoing management of [condition]."

If you have multiple objectives, it's often best to present your most pressing concern first. Once that has been addressed or acknowledged, you can then introduce secondary objectives. This structured approach helps maintain focus and ensure that the most critical issues are not overlooked. For example, you might say, "The main reason I wanted to see you today is because my knee pain has significantly worsened over the past week. I'm finding it difficult to walk. I also wanted to check in about my weight management goals and perhaps get a referral to a nutritionist." By clearly demarcating your primary concern, you guide the provider's attention effectively.

The preparation phase is crucial for defining and articulating these objectives. This might involve jotting down your concerns, symptoms, and questions in a notebook or on your smartphone in the days leading up to your appointment. This list serves as a personal reminder and a reference point during the consultation. When you arrive at the clinic, review your list and select your top one or two priorities for that visit. This structured approach helps to avoid feeling overwhelmed or forgetting important points in the moment.

It's also beneficial to consider the format of your objectives. Are there questions you need answered? Are there symptoms you need diagnosed? Are there treatment options you need discussed? Framing your objectives in a clear and actionable way will facilitate a more productive dialogue. For instance, instead of thinking, "I need to know about my heart," reframe it as a question or a specific concern: "I want to understand my recent ECG results and discuss what lifestyle changes I can make to improve my heart health."

When dealing with complex or multifaceted health issues, breaking down your overall health goals into smaller, manageable objectives for individual appointments can be very effective. For example, if your long-term goal is to achieve better overall cardiovascular health, your objectives for a series of visits might look like this:

Visit 1: Understand current risk factors (blood pressure, cholesterol, family history) and get baseline blood test results.

Visit 2: Discuss specific dietary changes recommended for heart health and clarify portion sizes and food choices.

Visit 3: Explore appropriate exercise regimens and set

realistic fitness goals.

Visit 4: Review progress, discuss any new symptoms or concerns, and adjust the plan as needed.

This step-by-step approach ensures that all aspects of your health concern are addressed systematically without overwhelming either you or the provider. It fosters a sense of progress and accomplishment along the way.

Furthermore, understanding the context of the visit can help you define your objectives. Is this a first-time visit for a new problem? A follow-up to monitor a chronic condition? A pre-operative assessment? A post-operative check-in? Each of these scenarios will naturally lead to different objectives. For a first-time visit for a specific symptom, the objective is likely diagnosis and initial treatment. For a chronic condition follow-up, it might be management optimization and monitoring. For pre-operative assessment, it's about ensuring you are fit for surgery and understanding the procedure. Tailoring your objectives to the specific purpose of the appointment makes your interaction more efficient and targeted.

It is also important to acknowledge that sometimes, the most crucial objective is simply to gain reassurance or to have your concerns validated. For patients experiencing anxiety about their health, or those who have felt dismissed in previous healthcare encounters, simply having their symptoms taken seriously and being provided with clear explanations can be a primary objective. If you feel your concerns are often minimized, you might state, "I've been quite worried about these symptoms, and I'd appreciate it if we could thoroughly discuss potential causes and rule out any serious conditions." This sets an expectation for a comprehensive and empathetic approach.

The ability to define and articulate health objectives is a skill that improves with practice. The more you engage in this process, the more adept you will become at identifying your needs and communicating them effectively. It empowers you as a patient, shifting you from a passive recipient of care to an active partner in your own health journey. This partnership is built on mutual understanding, clear communication, and shared goals, all of which are powerfully initiated by the simple yet profound act of defining your objectives before you even speak to your healthcare provider. It's about ensuring that every interaction moves you closer to your desired state of health and well-being, making the most of the invaluable time you spend with those dedicated to your care.

The foundation of a successful healthcare partnership rests on a crucial, often underestimated element: **trust.** Just as a strong marriage requires mutual faith and reliability, the relationship between a patient and their healthcare provider thrives on a shared sense of confidence, and mutual respect for each other's position. While providers are trained to foster an environment of trust, the patient also plays an indispensable role in its cultivation. This isn't about blind faith, but rather a conscious effort to build a bridge of understanding and reliance, ensuring that the journey towards optimal health is undertaken together, with both parties invested in the outcome.

Honesty, in its purest form, is the cornerstone of patient-provider trust. When you share your health information, whether it's about symptoms, lifestyle habits, or even personal history, it is imperative that this information be accurate and complete. This means being truthful about the onset and duration of symptoms, the medications you are taking (including over-the-counter drugs and supplements), your adherence to prescribed treatments, and any substances you may consume. Healthcare providers are not there to judge; they are there to help. Withholding or distorting information, even with the best intentions - perhaps to avoid embarrassment or a perceived lecture - can have significant, and sometimes dangerous, consequences. For instance, failing to mention that you occasionally skip doses of your blood pressure medication can lead the provider to believe the current dosage is ineffective, potentially resulting in an unnecessary increase that could cause side effects. Similarly, not disclosing your use of a particular herbal supplement might interfere with the efficacy or safety of a prescribed medication.

Consider a scenario where a patient is experiencing a persistent cough. They might feel embarrassed admitting to smoking, even though they know it's the likely culprit. If they omit this crucial detail, the provider might pursue extensive diagnostic tests, costing time, money, and causing unnecessary anxiety, all while the obvious cause remains unaddressed. The patient who is upfront about their smoking habit, however, allows the provider to immediately focus on smoking cessation strategies, which are far more likely to resolve the cough effectively and safely. A second scenario, I asked a patient if they had been drinking because it smelled like alcohol. However, he had diabetes, and I did not want to accuse him of drinking, and it was a ketoacidosis issue. I gave him a pain medication and he almost died, because he was not truthful with me. This level of honesty fosters an environment where the provider can make the most accurate assessments and tailor treatment plans that are genuinely beneficial. It's about providing the provider with all the pieces of the puzzle so they can see the complete picture and offer the best possible care.

Beyond medical information, honesty also extends to your expectations and understanding. If you don't understand a diagnosis, a treatment plan, or a recommendation, it is vital to voice that confusion. Pretending to comprehend when you don't create a gap in communication that can undermine trust.

A provider who believes you fully grasp the instructions might not offer further clarification, leading to potential misunderstandings and errors in care.

Expressing your uncertainties, such as saying, "I'm not sure I fully understand what this medication is for, or how it's supposed to help my condition," allows the provider to re-explain, offer alternative explanations, or provide written materials that can aid your comprehension. This open dialogue signals your engagement and your commitment to following through with the care plan.

Respecting the healthcare provider's expertise is another significant component of building trust. While you are the expert on your own body and experiences, your healthcare provider possesses specialized knowledge and training. Acknowledging and valuing this expertise, even when you have your own opinions or have done your own research (which is encouraged!), is crucial. This doesn't mean you should blindly accept every recommendation without question. It is healthy and appropriate to ask clarifying questions, seek second opinions, and engage in discussions about treatment options. However, it means approaching these discussions with an attitude of mutual respect, rather than adversarial confrontation.

When you present your research or concerns, frame them as collaborative points for discussion rather than definitive challenges to the provider's knowledge. For example, instead of stating, "My research shows that this alternative treatment is better than what you're recommending," a more trust-building approach would be: "I've been reading about [alternative treatment] and was wondering if it might be an option we could consider, or if you have any thoughts on its effectiveness compared to the current plan." This shows you've taken initiative in your health but are still seeking their professional guidance. It demonstrates that you value their opinion and are looking for their informed perspective.

Furthermore, respecting their time and the constraints of the healthcare system is also a demonstration of trust. Understanding that appointments have a set duration and that providers often manage a full schedule can help manage your own expectations and your approach to communication. Being prepared with your questions and objectives, as discussed in previous sections, allows for efficient use of the appointment time. It shows you respect the provider's commitment to serving other patients as well. Being punctual for appointments, arriving with necessary paperwork, and communicating any need to reschedule in a timely manner all contribute to a smoothly functioning partnership, reinforcing reliability.

A commitment to your own well-being, as demonstrated by your actions, is a powerful way to build trust. When a provider sees that you are actively engaged in managing your health, adhering to treatment plans, adopting healthier lifestyle choices, and taking recommended preventive measures, it reinforces their confidence in your commitment to your own care. This reciprocal investment makes the provider more likely to invest their time and expertise in your well-being. For instance, if you've been advised to increase your physical activity and you report on your progress, perhaps sharing that you've started walking three times a week, it shows you are taking their advice seriously. This kind of proactive engagement builds a positive feedback loop in the patient-provider relationship.

This commitment can manifest in various ways. It could be consistently attending follow-up appointments, diligently taking prescribed medications as directed, making necessary dietary changes, or engaging in recommended physical therapies. It also includes being proactive about your health beyond the doctor's office. This might involve learning more about your condition, utilizing patient portals to communicate with your care team, participating in health and wellness programs, or attending support groups. When you actively participate in managing your health, you are not just a recipient of care; you become a partner, demonstrating to your provider that you are a motivated and reliable participant in your own health journey. This shared commitment strengthens the bond of trust and encourages a more collaborative approach.

The development of trust is not an instantaneous event; it is a process that unfolds over time through consistent, positive interactions. Each honest conversation, each shared moment of understanding, and each step taken towards better health, collectively builds this vital foundation. It requires effort from both sides, but by understanding and embracing your role in cultivating trust, you empower yourself to build a stronger, more effective, and ultimately more rewarding healthcare partnership. This partnership is not just about receiving treatment; it is about shared responsibility, mutual respect, and a unified effort to achieve the best possible health outcomes.

2: Mastering Symptom Articulation and Communication

The ability to articulate your symptoms with precision is akin to a skilled artist's brushstrokes, where each detail contributes to a clearer, more accurate picture. Simply stating "I have pain" is a starting point, but it's the nuanced description that unlocks the diagnostic potential for your healthcare provider. Think of yourself as a detective presenting clues; the more specific and organized your evidence, the faster and more accurately the case can be solved. This subsection delves into the art of symptom description, transforming a general complaint into actionable information.

When discussing pain, a range of descriptors is invaluable. Instead of just saying it hurts, consider the *quality* of the pain. Is it a dull ache, a sharp stab, a burning sensation, a throbbing, or a gnawing discomfort? Each of these words evokes a different physiological response and can point towards different underlying causes. A burning pain, for example, might suggest nerve involvement or an inflammatory process, while a dull ache could be muscular or skeletal in origin. Likewise, describing pain as constricting, cramping, or tearing provides further vital clues. For instance, a constricting chest pain might raise concerns about cardiac issues, whereas a cramping sensation in the abdomen could indicate gastrointestinal distress. A sharp, sudden pain is often perceived differently by the body than a persistent, throbbing discomfort, and communicating these nuances is crucial for the provider's differential diagnosis.

The *intensity* of the pain is another critical piece of information. While subjective, using a pain scale can standardize this. The common 0-10 scale, where 0 is no pain and 10 is the worst imaginable pain, allows you to quantify your experience. When you report a pain level of, say, 7 out of 10, it gives the provider a benchmark. It's also helpful to describe how this intensity fluctuates. Does it remain at a constant 7, or does it surge to an 8 or 9 at times? Does it ever dip to a 3 or 4? Understanding this variability can reveal patterns related to activity, rest, or medication. For example, pain that spikes to an 8 after walking but returns to a 4 at rest suggests a mechanical or musculoskeletal origin, whereas pain that stays at a consistent 6 throughout the day might indicate a more chronic or systemic issue.

The *location* of the pain, and whether it radiates, is equally important. Be as specific as possible. Is the pain localized to a small, pinpoint area, or is it diffuse across a larger region? For instance, stating "pain in my lower back" is helpful, but specifying "pain on the right side of my lower back, about the size of a quarter, that sometimes shoots down my leg" provides much more diagnostic direction. Radiation of pain, often described as "shooting," "traveling," or "radiating," is a key indicator of nerve compression or irritation. Knowing precisely where the pain originates and where it travels helps pinpoint the affected anatomical structures. If pain originates in the shoulder and radiates down the arm, it suggests different possibilities than pain that is confined to the shoulder joint itself. Similarly, abdominal pain that radiates to the back can be a sign of pancreatic issues, while pain in the upper abdomen that radiates to the jaw might suggest a cardiac event.

Beyond pain, describing other symptoms requires a similar level of detail. For *fatigue*, for instance, it's not just about feeling tired. Is it a profound lack of energy that prevents you from performing daily tasks? Does it feel like overwhelming sleepiness, or a mental fogginess that makes concentration difficult? Is the fatigue constant, or does it worsen at particular times of the day? Does it improve with rest, or does rest offer no relief? For example, fatigue that is worse in the morning and improves as the day goes on might be related to sleep disorders, while fatigue that is persistent and exacerbated by activity could point to a more systemic illness.

When describing *digestive issues,* specificity is paramount. Instead of saying "stomach problems," consider details like the frequency and nature of nausea, vomiting, diarrhea, or constipation. What is the consistency of the stool? Is there blood or mucus present? Is the discomfort related to eating? For example, nausea that occurs immediately after eating might suggest gastritis or peptic ulcer disease, while diarrhea that occurs several hours after meals could indicate food intolerance or malabsorption issues. The presence of blood in the stool, whether bright red or dark and tarry, is always a significant symptom that requires immediate attention and detailed description of its appearance and frequency.

For *respiratory symptoms,* such as cough or shortness of breath, detail is critical. What is the nature of the cough? Is it dry and hacking, or is it productive, bringing up phlegm? If productive, what is the color and consistency of the phlegm? Is there any blood? How severe is the shortness of breath? Does it occur with exertion, at rest, or when lying down? For example, a dry, ticklish cough might be due to allergies or irritation, while a deep, rattling cough with thick, colored phlegm suggests an infection like bronchitis or pneumonia. Shortness of breath that is worse when lying flat (orthopnea) is a classic sign of heart failure.

The *duration* and *frequency* of symptoms are also essential components of accurate description. How long has the symptom been present? Did it start suddenly, or has it developed gradually over weeks or months? How often does the symptom occur? Is it constant, intermittent, or does it happen only under specific circumstances? For instance, a headache that has been present for a week is different from a headache that occurs daily. A rash that appears and disappears is different from a rash that is persistently present. Understanding the timeline helps the provider differentiate between acute and chronic conditions. Is the symptom a new occurrence or a recurrence of a previous issue? If it is a recurrence, how does this episode compare to previous ones?

Furthermore, identifying *associated factors* or *triggers* can provide significant diagnostic clues. What makes the symptom worse? What makes it better? Are there specific foods, activities, medications, or environmental factors that seem to precede the onset or exacerbation of the symptom? For example, if a rash appears after exposure to sunlight, it suggests a photosensitivity reaction. If joint pain worsens in cold weather, it might indicate arthritis. If a symptom improves after taking a particular medication, it can offer insight into its nature. Documenting these associations, even if they seem minor or coincidental, is incredibly valuable. It is also important to note if any symptoms occur in clusters or sequences. Does the headache always precede the nausea, or does the dizziness occur after the chest tightness?

The *timing* of symptoms can also be revealing. Do symptoms occur at a particular time of day or night? For example, symptoms of asthma often worsen at night, while symptoms of gastroesophageal reflux disease (GERD) might be more pronounced after meals or when lying down. Morning stiffness in joints can be indicative of inflammatory arthritis, while stiffness that improves with activity might suggest osteoarthritis.

When describing symptoms, it is also helpful to consider the *impact* the symptom is having on your daily life. Is it interfering with your work, sleep, social activities, or ability to care for yourself or others? This provides context for the severity of the symptom and helps the provider understand the burden of your condition. For example, knowing that fatigue prevents you from working or that pain limits your mobility helps the provider prioritize treatment goals.

To effectively gather and present this detailed information, keeping a symptom journal can be immensely beneficial. Before your appointment, take some time to jot down your symptoms using the descriptors discussed above. Note the date and time each symptom occurred, its characteristics, intensity, duration, location, radiation, associated factors, and any treatments you tried and their effects. This structured approach ensures that you don't forget crucial details in the stress of a medical consultation. It also serves as a reference point for tracking changes in your condition over time.

Consider the difference between saying "I feel dizzy" and saying "I experienced a sudden spinning sensation (vertigo) that lasted for about a minute this morning after I stood up too quickly. It made me feel like I was going to fall, but it resolved on its own. I haven't had it since, but I feel a bit unsteady." The second description provides specific information about the type of dizziness (vertigo), its onset, duration, triggering factor, severity, and resolution, which are all critical for diagnosis.

Another example: a patient might say, "I have a cough." A more detailed description would be: "I've had a cough for about two weeks. It's mostly dry, but sometimes I bring up a little clear phlegm. It's worse at night and when I lie down, and it sometimes wakes me up. It doesn't feel like it's related to exertion or any specific food. I haven't had a fever, but I do feel a bit more tired than usual." This level of detail helps the provider consider various causes, from post-viral irritation to early signs of bronchitis or even something more serious like a lung condition, and it guides their subsequent questions and examination.

The importance of providing this granular detail cannot be overstated. It's not about overwhelming your provider with information, but about providing them with the most relevant and accurate data points. When you can describe your symptoms with clarity and precision, you empower your healthcare provider to make more informed decisions, leading to a more efficient and effective diagnostic process and, ultimately, a better treatment plan tailored specifically to your needs. This meticulous approach transforms you from a passive recipient of care into an active, informed participant in your own health journey, laying the groundwork for a truly collaborative partnership.

Remember, your healthcare provider relies on your description to form hypotheses about what might be happening. Vague or incomplete information can lead them down the wrong diagnostic path, delaying effective treatment and potentially causing unnecessary anxiety and expense. By mastering the art of symptom articulation, you are essentially providing the essential ingredients for an accurate diagnosis and a successful therapeutic outcome. This skill is as fundamental to receiving good healthcare as the provider's expertise itself. It is an investment in clarity, accuracy, and ultimately, in your own well-being.

The intricate dance of a healthcare interaction extends far beyond the spoken word. While articulating your symptoms with precision is paramount, the silent language of non-verbal communication plays an equally vital role in conveying your health status and concerns to your healthcare provider. These subtle cues—your posture, facial expressions, eye contact, and even the cadence of your voice—can powerfully amplify or, conversely, muddle the message you intend to send. Developing an awareness of these non-verbal signals, both your own and those of your provider, can significantly enhance the clarity and effectiveness of your dialogue, fostering a deeper understanding and a more collaborative approach to your care.

Consider, for instance, the message conveyed by your posture. Arriving at an appointment slumped in your chair, with shoulders rounded and head bowed, can immediately signal fatigue, pain, or a general sense of disengagement, even before you utter a word. Conversely, sitting upright, perhaps leaning slightly forward, can communicate attentiveness and a proactive engagement with the consultation. If you are experiencing physical discomfort that limits your ability to sit or stand in certain ways, this is also a non-verbal cue. Perhaps you shift frequently in your seat, or you unconsciously cradle a specific part of your body where you feel pain. These are not simply random movements; they are often unconscious expressions of your internal state. For example, a patient with significant back pain might struggle to sit still for an extended period, constantly adjusting their position to find a less painful stance. This physical manifestation of discomfort, without them needing to explicitly state the degree of their pain at that very moment, is a powerful piece of information for a discerning healthcare provider. Similarly, if a patient is experiencing shortness of breath, their posture might reflect this—perhaps sitting forward, using their hands to support themselves, or even exhibiting a shallow, rapid breathing pattern that is visible. These are all non-verbal communications that add layers to the spoken narrative.

Facial expressions are another incredibly potent channel of non-verbal communication. A furrowed brow can indicate worry or confusion, while a strained smile might suggest discomfort masked by an effort to appear stoic. A grimace of pain, even if brief, is unmistakable. Conversely, an open, relaxed expression can convey a sense of well-being or a readiness to communicate. Think about how easily we interpret a child's tear-streaked face and downturned mouth as sadness or pain. The same principle applies in the clinical setting. Even if you say, "I'm feeling okay," a wince when you attempt to move a painful limb speaks volumes more about your true physical state. It's about congruence: when your verbal and non-verbal messages align, your communication is clear and credible. When they are incongruent—for example, saying you are not experiencing pain while your facial muscles are visibly tensed and your eyes are squeezed shut—your provider is likely to trust the non-verbal cues more, as they are often more difficult to consciously control. The subtle tightening around the eyes during a sharp pain, the slight puffing of cheeks during labored breathing, or the involuntary clenching of the jaw during intense discomfort are all signals that a provider trained in observation will pick up.

The act of making eye contact, or the lack thereof, also carries significant weight. Direct eye contact typically signifies engagement, honesty, and confidence. Avoiding eye contact can sometimes be interpreted as evasiveness, discomfort, or even deception, although it's crucial to remember that cultural norms and individual personality traits can heavily influence this. For someone with social anxiety or certain neurodevelopmental conditions, avoiding eye contact might be a coping mechanism, not an indicator of dishonesty. Therefore, it's important to consider the broader context. However, in the general sense, maintaining appropriate eye contact with your provider demonstrates that you are present and actively participating in the conversation. If you find yourself unable to make sustained eye contact due to discomfort or anxiety, a brief acknowledgment of this—"I'm finding it hard to make eye contact right now because I'm feeling very anxious about this"—can pre-empt misinterpretation.

Your tone of voice, even more than the words you choose, can convey the emotional undertone of your experience. A shaky voice might suggest fear or anxiety. A flat, monotone delivery could indicate profound fatigue or depression. Conversely, a clear, steady voice can project confidence and clarity. Consider the difference between saying "I'm feeling tired" in a weak, breathy voice versus saying it in a strong, measured tone. The former conveys a deeper level of exhaustion or illness, while the latter might simply be stating a fact. The pitch, volume, and speed of your speech are all non-verbal elements that contribute to the overall message. For example, a patient describing debilitating pain might speak in short, clipped sentences, with a higher pitch due to tension, and a noticeable pause between phrases as they gather breath or cope with the discomfort. This contrasts with a patient describing a mild, intermittent symptom who might speak in a more relaxed, fluid manner. Even if the words used to describe the symptom are similar, the vocal delivery provides crucial additional information about the severity and impact of the condition.

Moreover, gestures and touch can communicate important information. Fidgeting might indicate nervousness or discomfort. A hand repeatedly touching a painful area is a direct, non-verbal pointer to the source of distress. If you are experiencing nausea, you might unconsciously press a hand to your abdomen or stomach. If you have a headache, you might rub your temples. These are universally understood gestures of discomfort or pain. When a provider asks you to describe the location of your pain, and you point directly to a specific spot, that physical gesture is an immediate and effective form of communication. Similarly, if a provider is examining a tender area, your involuntary flinching or sharp intake of breath is a powerful non-verbal response that communicates the presence and intensity of pain.

Being aware of your own non-verbal signals is the first step in leveraging them effectively. Before your appointment, take a moment to consider how you typically present yourself when you are unwell. Are you generally withdrawn? Do you tend to minimize your symptoms, even non-verbally? Practicing articulating your symptoms in front of a mirror can help you observe your own facial expressions and body language. This self-awareness allows you to consciously project a more open and communicative demeanor, even when you are feeling vulnerable. It might involve reminding yourself to sit up straight, to take deep breaths if you feel anxious, or to try and maintain eye contact as much as is comfortable.

Equally important is the ability to interpret the non-verbal cues of your healthcare providers. While their primary role is to listen to your words, their own body language can offer insights. Is the provider leaning in, appearing engaged, or are they frequently glancing at their watch or computer screen, appearing distracted? Do they maintain eye contact when you are speaking, or do they seem preoccupied? A provider who nods along, maintains eye contact, and occasionally uses encouraging gestures like a gentle pat on the arm (if appropriate and culturally sensitive) is conveying attentiveness and empathy. Conversely, a provider who seems rushed, interrupts frequently, or displays closed-off body language (crossed arms, avoiding eye contact) might be perceived as less approachable, potentially making you feel less comfortable sharing sensitive information.

However, it is vital to avoid making definitive judgments based solely on non-verbal cues. Healthcare professionals are human beings with their own potential stressors, time constraints, and communication styles. A provider who appears distracted might be managing a complex medical emergency happening elsewhere, or they might simply be a naturally reserved individual. The key is to observe these cues, consider them as part of the overall interaction, but not let them solely dictate your perception of the care you are receiving. If you feel unheard or disconnected due to perceived non-verbal signals, it is often more productive to address this directly and constructively. You could say something like, "I'm feeling a little concerned that I might not be explaining this clearly. Is there anything I can do to help you understand what I'm experiencing?" or "I'm finding it a bit difficult to convey how much this symptom is affecting me. Could we perhaps spend a few more minutes on this aspect?" This approach opens the door for clarification without making accusations.

The environment of the consultation also influences non-verbal communication. A quiet, private room allows for more open and honest exchange than a busy, noisy waiting area. The physical space between you and your provider can also play a role. Too close, and it might feel intrusive; too far, and it might feel distant. A provider who positions themselves at a comfortable distance, perhaps sitting at eye level with you rather than standing over you, helps to create a more balanced and respectful dynamic.

Consider a scenario where a patient is describing a symptom that causes them significant embarrassment or shame, such as incontinence or a sexual health issue. Their non-verbal cues—a tendency to whisper, avoid eye contact, cross their arms tightly, or blush—will likely be pronounced. A sensitive provider will recognize these signals and respond with reassurance, a calm demeanor, and a focus on creating a safe space for disclosure. They might say, "Thank you for sharing this with me. Many people find these issues difficult to talk about, and I want you to know that we can discuss this openly and confidentially." This verbal reassurance, coupled with gentle, professional non-verbal cues, can help alleviate the patient's distress and facilitate open communication.

Another example could involve a patient with chronic pain who has learned to mask their discomfort through outward signs of normalcy. They might force a smile, maintain a steady gaze, and speak in an even tone, all while experiencing significant internal distress.

However, subtle non-verbal cues might still betray their true state: a slight tremor in their hands, a fleeting grimace that they quickly suppress, or a particular stiffness in their movements that they try to disguise. A perceptive provider might pick up on these inconsistencies and gently probe further, perhaps by asking, "You're presenting a very strong face, which I appreciate, but I sense there might be more going on. How are you truly feeling right now, beyond the stoicism?" This allows the patient an opening to drop their guard and express their genuine experience.

The integration of verbal and non-verbal communication is what creates a holistic understanding. When your words describe a specific type of pain, and your facial expression matches that description—perhaps a pained grimace for sharp pain, or a look of weariness for dull, persistent ache—your communication is exceptionally clear. If you describe feeling anxious, and your voice trembles slightly, your body language is tense, and your breath is shallow, the message is powerfully reinforced.

This congruence between what you say and how you say it (and how you appear) builds trust and confidence in the provider's understanding of your situation.

As a patient advocate, it is important to encourage individuals to harness the power of their own non-verbal signals. This isn't about putting on a performance, but about ensuring that your internal experience is accurately reflected externally. If you are feeling particularly unwell, it is perfectly acceptable to appear so. Your provider needs to see and understand the impact your symptoms are having. Holding back tears when discussing a distressing symptom, for instance, is a natural expression of your emotional state and can be a vital communication tool, conveying the depth of your suffering more effectively than words alone. Similarly, if you are experiencing a symptom that causes physical distress when you move, such as dizziness or joint pain, allowing your provider to observe this naturally occurring reaction during an examination is far more informative than simply describing it.

Furthermore, recognizing that your non-verbal cues can influence your provider's perception of your credibility and your commitment to your health is important. Someone who appears engaged, attentive, and proactive in their communication—through their posture, eye contact, and vocal tone—is often perceived as someone who is taking their health seriously. This can, in turn, foster a more collaborative and respectful relationship with their healthcare team.

The art of effective communication in healthcare is thus a dual process: mastering the articulation of your symptoms and becoming attuned to the silent language that accompanies them. By paying attention to your own body language, facial expressions, and tone of voice, and by learning to interpret those of your healthcare provider, you can build stronger bridges of understanding. This awareness transforms your interactions from potentially transactional exchanges into truly collaborative partnerships, where every cue, spoken or unspoken, contributes to a clearer, more accurate picture of your health. It empowers you to advocate for your needs more effectively and ensures that your experience is understood in its entirety, paving the way for the most appropriate and compassionate care. This deeper level of connection, built on both verbal clarity and non-verbal understanding, is fundamental to navigating the complexities of the healthcare system with confidence and ensuring that your journey towards wellness is as well-supported as possible. It's about recognizing that in the intricate tapestry of a doctor-patient relationship, every thread counts, and the silent threads of non-verbal communication are often among the most revealing and impactful.

The journey toward truly mastering symptom articulation and effective communication with your healthcare team is significantly bolstered by the diligent use of specific tools designed to capture and organize your health experiences.

Among the most powerful of these are symptom journals and health logs. These are not merely diaries of daily occurrences; rather, they are meticulously crafted records that serve as a comprehensive, objective repository of your symptoms, their evolution, and their impact on your life. By committing to keeping such a record, you transform yourself from a passive observer of your own health into an active participant in its management, equipped with data that is invaluable to your clinician.

Think of a symptom journal as your personal health narrative, penned with the precision of a scientific observer. Its primary purpose is to provide a clear, chronological account of your symptoms, moving beyond the often-fragmented recall that occurs when asked about them during a brief appointment. The effectiveness of this tool lies in its ability to capture nuances that might otherwise be forgotten or downplayed. When you sit down to write, you are prompted to consider specific aspects of your experience, forcing a deeper level of introspection and detail. For instance, rather than simply stating "I have a headache," a journal entry might read: "August 15th, 8:00 AM: Migraine-type headache started upon waking. Located behind left eye, throbbing. Intensity 7/10. Accompanied by nausea and sensitivity to light.

Took 400mg ibuprofen at 8:30 AM. Slight relief by 9:30 AM, intensity reduced to 5/10. Avoided bright lights and noise. Able to function but with significant discomfort. No clear trigger identified yesterday, but sleep was disrupted." This level of detail is a goldmine for a healthcare provider, offering a clear picture of the symptom's characteristics, severity, response to treatment, and its impact on your daily activities.

The practical application of a symptom journal

begins with its format. There is no single prescribed method; the best approach is one that you can consistently maintain. Some individuals prefer a traditional pen-and-paper notebook, appreciating the tactile experience and the sense of permanence it offers. Others find digital solutions more convenient, utilizing dedicated health apps or even a simple spreadsheet or word document on their phone or computer. Regardless of the medium, the key is to establish a routine for recording your symptoms. This might mean dedicating a few minutes each evening to jot down any significant health events of the day, or perhaps making it a habit to update your journal immediately after experiencing a new or worsening symptom. Consistency is paramount; sporadic entries will diminish the journal's utility.

When beginning to keep a symptom journal, it's helpful to consider the key categories of information that will make your entries most informative. These typically include:

Date and Time: Precise timing helps to identify patterns and track symptom duration.

Symptom Description: Be specific. Instead of "pain,"

describe the quality of the pain (sharp, dull, aching, burning, throbbing), its location (e.g., "upper right abdomen," "left shoulder blade"), and its intensity. Using a rating scale, such as 0-10, where 0 is no pain and 10 is the worst imaginable, can provide a standardized measure of severity.

Onset: When did the symptom begin? Was it sudden or gradual?

Triggers: What factors appeared to precede or exacerbate the symptom? This could include specific foods, activities, environmental conditions (e.g., heat, cold, noise), stress levels, or even the time of day. Identifying triggers is crucial for management strategies. For example, noting that a particular type of meal consistently leads to indigestion provides actionable information for dietary changes.

Relieving Factors: What actions or interventions lessened the symptom? This includes medications (specifying the type, dosage, and time taken), rest, specific positions, heat or cold application, or other self-care measures.

Associated Symptoms: Are there other symptoms that occur alongside the primary one? For example, a headache might be accompanied by nausea, dizziness, or visual disturbances.

Impact on Daily Life: How does the symptom affect your ability to perform everyday activities? This could include work, sleep, exercise, social interactions, or personal care. Quantifying this impact, such as "unable to work for two days due to fatigue" or "difficulty climbing stairs because of shortness of breath," offers a clear picture of the symptom's burden.

Duration: How long did the symptom last?

Any Changes or Observations: This is a catch-all for anything else you deem relevant, such as changes in appetite, mood, energy levels, or any new or unusual sensations.

Let's explore this with a more detailed example. Imagine a patient experiencing persistent fatigue. A simple note in their journal might be "August 10th: Very tired today." However, a more effective entry would look like this:

"August 10th, 7:00 AM: Woke up feeling exhausted, slept for 9 hours but did not feel rested. Fatigue intensity 8/10. Difficulty concentrating at work by 9:30 AM.

Experienced a brief period of increased energy after lunch (around 1:00 PM), but it subsided within an hour. Did not engage in strenuous activity yesterday. Last night's dinner was a heavy meal around 7:00 PM. Evening fatigue intensity 7/10. Felt too tired to engage in social activities. Tried a 30-minute nap at 4:00 PM, which provided minimal relief."

This entry provides a wealth of information: the quality of the fatigue (unrested waking, fluctuating energy), its severity, its impact on cognitive function, potential timing of improvements, relationship to recent activity and diet, and its effect on social engagement. When presented with such a detailed log, a healthcare provider can begin to formulate hypotheses about the underlying causes. Is this fatigue related to sleep apnea, anemia, a thyroid condition, depression, or an autoimmune disorder? The journal entry helps to narrow down the possibilities and guides the diagnostic process.

Beyond the detailed symptom journal, a broader health log can also be incredibly beneficial. This might encompass not just symptoms, but also vital signs (if you monitor them at home, such as blood pressure or blood glucose), medication adherence, appointment dates and outcomes, and even significant lifestyle changes or stressors. A comprehensive health log can paint a more complete picture of your overall health status and how various factors interact. For instance, tracking your blood pressure alongside your symptom entries might reveal a correlation between elevated readings and the onset of certain symptoms like headaches or dizziness.

Similarly, noting when you missed a dose of medication and observing any subsequent changes in your symptoms can highlight the importance of adherence.

The benefits of maintaining these records extend beyond simply providing information to your doctor. The act of journaling itself can be therapeutic, offering a sense of control and understanding over your health conditions. It encourages mindfulness, prompting you to pay closer attention to your body's signals and how they respond to different interventions. This heightened self-awareness can lead to earlier recognition of symptom changes, allowing for prompt medical attention and potentially preventing more serious complications. Furthermore, by having a documented history, you are less likely to feel dismissed or misunderstood if your symptoms fluctuate or if you encounter different healthcare providers. Your journal becomes your voice, providing consistent and reliable information even when you are feeling unwell or struggling to articulate your experiences.

When presenting your journal or log to your healthcare provider, it's useful to be prepared. Before your appointment, review your entries to identify the most important points you want to convey. You might even want to create a brief summary of your key concerns or trends observed in your log. For instance, you could say, "I've been keeping this journal of my headaches, and I've noticed they seem to be worse on days when I have less than six hours of sleep and consume caffeine after noon. I also want to discuss the nausea that accompanies them." This concise summary, supported by the detailed records, ensures that your most pressing issues are addressed efficiently.

It is also important to discuss with your provider how they would prefer to receive this information. Some may be happy to review a physical notebook or a printed digital log, while others might prefer access to a specific app or a digital file. Open communication about your record-keeping practices fosters a collaborative approach. If your provider suggests a different way of tracking information, be open to incorporating their suggestions, as they may have insights into what is most valuable from a clinical perspective.

In essence, symptom journals and health logs empower you to be an active and informed participant in your healthcare journey. They provide the objective data needed for accurate diagnosis and effective treatment, while also fostering a deeper understanding of your own body. By consistently and thoughtfully documenting your experiences, you equip yourself and your healthcare team with the essential tools for navigating your health challenges with clarity and confidence. This practice transforms communication from a reactive, potentially unreliable exchange into a proactive, data-driven dialogue, paving the way for more personalized and effective care. The commitment to this practice is an investment in your well-being, ensuring that every facet of your health experience is seen, understood, and acted upon.

The journey of managing your health is significantly enhanced when you move beyond passive reception of medical advice and actively engage in dialogue with your healthcare providers. This engagement is not simply about voicing concerns, but about asking the *right* questions—questions that illuminate, clarify, and empower you to make informed decisions about your well-being. Developing this skill transforms your interactions from one-sided consultations into collaborative partnerships, where your understanding and participation are paramount.

Consider your appointment as an opportunity to gather crucial intelligence about your health. Before you even set foot in the clinic, it's beneficial to prepare a list of questions. This preparation can stem directly from the notes you've diligently kept in your symptom journal or health log. Perhaps you've identified a new symptom that puzzles you, a change in an existing one that concerns you, or a lack of response to a prescribed treatment. These observations are the bedrock upon which effective questions are built. For instance, if your journal indicates a persistent, unexplained fatigue that is impacting your work and personal life, your initial question might be straightforward: "I've been experiencing significant fatigue for the past few weeks, and it's affecting my ability to concentrate and complete daily tasks. Could we explore potential causes for this?" This opening statement is clear, states the problem, and directly asks for an investigation.

When your doctor provides a diagnosis, it's natural to feel a mix of emotions, which can sometimes make it difficult to absorb information. This is where well-formulated questions become indispensable. Instead of simply nodding in understanding, consider digging deeper. After hearing a diagnosis, you might ask: "Could you please explain what this diagnosis means in simpler terms? What are the primary mechanisms causing this condition?" Understanding the "what" and the "why" behind your diagnosis is fundamental. Following this, a crucial question is about the certainty of the diagnosis: "How confident are you in this diagnosis, and are there any other conditions that present with similar symptoms that we should consider or rule out?" This question acknowledges that medical diagnoses can sometimes be complex and may require further investigation, demonstrating your engagement with the diagnostic process and your desire for accuracy.

Once a diagnosis is established, the focus naturally shifts to treatment. Here, the goal is to understand your options, their benefits, and their drawbacks. Begin by asking about the recommended course of action: "What is the recommended treatment plan for this condition?" This opens the door to a discussion about specific therapies, medications, or lifestyle changes. However, a truly empowered patient will then probe further into the alternatives. "Are there other treatment options available besides the one you're suggesting? What are the pros and cons of each option?" This demonstrates your interest in exploring the full spectrum of possibilities and weighing them according to your personal circumstances and values. For example, if a medication is prescribed, you might ask about its mechanism of action, its expected timeline for effectiveness, and what to do if it doesn't seem to be working.

Understanding the rationale behind the treatment plan—how it works and what results to anticipate—is vital for adherence and managing expectations.

A critical aspect of any treatment is understanding potential side effects. It is not enough to be told there "might be side effects." Specificity is key. You should ask: "What are the most common side effects associated with this treatment, and how should I manage them if they occur?" Moreover, it's important to inquire about less common but potentially serious side effects: "Are there any rare but serious side effects I should be aware of, and what symptoms would necessitate immediate medical attention?" This proactive approach to side effect management can prevent undue alarm and ensure you know when to seek help. For instance, if you are prescribed a new medication, you might ask, "Should I expect any immediate side effects after taking the first dose, or do they tend to develop over time?" or "Are there any specific interactions I should be aware of with other medications I'm currently taking, or even with over-the-counter supplements or foods?" Providing your doctor with a comprehensive list of everything you consume, including vitamins, herbal remedies, and even recreational substances, will enable them to give you the most accurate advice regarding potential interactions.

Beyond the immediate treatment, understanding the long-term outlook, or prognosis, is also essential. This involves asking about the expected course of the condition and the goals of treatment. "What is the expected outcome of this treatment, and what is the long-term prognosis for this condition?" you might inquire. "Is the goal of treatment to cure the condition, manage its symptoms, or slow its progression?" Clarifying the objectives helps you understand what success looks like and what to anticipate in the months and years ahead. You might also ask about lifestyle modifications that can support recovery or improve the prognosis: "Are there specific lifestyle changes, such as diet or exercise, that could significantly impact my recovery or the long-term management of this condition?" This moves the conversation towards a holistic view of your health, recognizing that medical treatments are often most effective when complemented by personal health behaviors.

When discussing treatment plans, particularly those involving surgery or complex procedures, it's wise to understand the alternatives and the risks involved. "What are the risks associated with this procedure, and how do they compare to the risks of not having the procedure?" is a fundamental question. You might also ask about the success rates of the procedure, the typical recovery period, and what to expect during the healing process. "How long is the typical recovery period, and what level of activity can I expect to resume and when?" Understanding the rehabilitation process, including any physical therapy or follow-up care, sets realistic expectations and helps you prepare for the recovery phase.

It's also important to ask about follow-up appointments and monitoring. "How will my progress be monitored, and when should I schedule my next appointment?" This ensures that your care is a continuous process and that your healthcare team remains involved in tracking your response to treatment and managing any evolving issues.

Knowing when and how to check in can prevent the sense of being "finished" with care after an initial consultation and reinforce the ongoing nature of health management.

For those managing chronic conditions, the

questions evolve to focus on self-management and long-term quality of life. "What are the warning signs that my condition is worsening or that my current treatment is no longer effective?" is a vital question for maintaining vigilance. Furthermore, understanding how your condition might interact with other aspects of your life is important: "How might this condition affect my ability to travel, work, or engage in my hobbies, and are there strategies to mitigate these impacts?" This broadens the scope of the conversation to encompass your overall well-being and life satisfaction.

Remember, your healthcare provider is a resource, but they cannot read your mind or intuit your deepest concerns. Taking the initiative to ask questions is not a sign of distrust, but a mark of an engaged and informed patient. It demonstrates respect for your own health and a commitment to actively participating in your care. Sometimes, the act of asking a question, even if the answer is something you already suspected, can bring a sense of validation and clarity. It solidifies your understanding and reinforces the shared responsibility for your health outcomes.

To facilitate this questioning process, consider using a structured approach during your appointment. After the doctor has explained the diagnosis and proposed a treatment plan, you could systematically go through categories of questions:

1. **Diagnosis Clarification:** "Can you explain that again, perhaps using a different analogy?" or "What does this diagnosis mean for my body specifically?"

2. **Treatment Options:** "What are the goals of this treatment? Are there non-medicinal approaches we should consider first?"

3. **Medication Details (if applicable):** "How and when should I take this medication? What should I do if I miss a dose? What are the most common side effects, and what are the signs of a serious reaction?"

4. **Prognosis and Long-Term Outlook:** "What is the typical course of this condition? Will this treatment cure it or manage it? What does a successful outcome look like in the long term?"

5. **Lifestyle and Self-Care:** "What dietary changes or physical activities would be most beneficial? Are there any I should avoid?"

6. **Follow-Up and Monitoring:** "How will we track my progress? When should I expect to see improvements? What signs indicate I need to contact you before my next scheduled appointment?"

By organizing your inquiries, you ensure that no critical area is overlooked. It also provides a clear structure for your doctor to address each of your concerns comprehensively. Don't be afraid to ask for clarification if an answer is still unclear. Phrases like "I'm still not quite understanding this..." or "Could you elaborate on that point?" are perfectly acceptable and encourage further explanation.

It's also valuable to ask about your role in your own recovery and management. "What specific actions can I take between appointments to improve my health or manage my symptoms?" This empowers you to be an active agent in your care, fostering a sense of control and responsibility. Questions about preventive measures for the future are also important: "Are there any steps I can take to reduce the risk of this condition recurring or worsening?" or "Are there any lifestyle changes that can support long-term health and well-being related to this condition?"

In some instances, you may feel that your questions haven't been fully addressed or that you need more information. In such cases, it's perfectly reasonable to ask, "Is there anything else I should know about this diagnosis or treatment that we haven't discussed?" or "Would it be helpful for me to schedule a follow-up call with the nurse or a medical assistant to clarify these points?" Some healthcare systems offer patient education resources or support groups that could be beneficial, so inquiring about these can also be a valuable part of your information-gathering process.

Finally, remember that your relationship with your healthcare provider is built on trust and open communication. Asking questions is a fundamental way to build and maintain that trust. It signals that you are invested in your health and that you are a partner in the decision-making process. By preparing thoughtful questions and engaging actively in your consultations, you not only gain a deeper understanding of your health but also contribute significantly to the effectiveness of your care. This proactive approach ensures that you are not merely a recipient of medical services, but a well-informed advocate for your own well-being.

When the landscape of your health journey presents challenging terrain, it's not uncommon to encounter situations that require navigating conversations that feel inherently difficult. These are the discussions that might involve sensitive personal information, complex medical jargon that's hard to grasp, or deeply rooted anxieties about a diagnosis or treatment plan. The very nature of illness can make us vulnerable, and articulating our deepest fears or the most nuanced of our physical sensations can feel like an overwhelming task, especially when speaking with a medical professional whose expertise is so vital. Yet, it is precisely in these moments of discomfort that the ability to communicate effectively becomes paramount.

Mastering these difficult conversations isn't about confronting or challenging your healthcare provider; rather, it's about fostering a deeper, more collaborative relationship built on mutual understanding and a shared commitment to your well-being. It's about ensuring that your voice, your experiences, and your emotional state are fully heard and integrated into your care plan.

One of the primary hurdles in these conversations is the sheer emotional weight that can accompany them. Receiving a diagnosis, particularly one that is serious or life-altering, can trigger a cascade of emotions: fear, anger, sadness, confusion, or even disbelief. In the face of such emotional intensity, the ability to articulate symptoms or concerns can feel severely compromised. It's as if a fog descends, making it difficult to recall the precise details of your physical experience or to frame your questions coherently. To counter this, remember the preparatory work you've done—your symptom journal. This log is not just a record of physical manifestations; it's also a repository of your evolving understanding and emotional responses. Before an appointment where you anticipate a difficult discussion, revisit your journal. Note down not only the symptoms but also any thoughts or feelings that have accompanied them. For example, if you've been diagnosed with a chronic condition that impacts your mobility, your journal might detail not just the physical pain or stiffness, but also the frustration of not being able to participate in activities you once enjoyed, or the fear of becoming a burden. When you enter the consultation room, you can use these notes as anchors. Instead of trying to recall everything at once, you can say, "I've been feeling increasingly anxious about how my condition is affecting my ability to walk my dog, as noted in my journal. It's not just the physical discomfort, but the fear of falling that really concerns me." This approach grounds your emotional state in tangible experiences, making it easier for your healthcare provider to understand the full scope of your concerns.

Another aspect of difficult conversations involves seeking clarity on complex medical information. Healthcare providers often operate within a framework of specialized knowledge, using terminology that is precise for them but opaque to patients. When faced with a diagnosis or a treatment plan that is explained using technical language, it is essential to ask for simplification without feeling embarrassed or unintelligent.

The key is to frame your request for clarification positively and proactively. Instead of saying, "I don't understand anything you're saying," which can sound confrontational, try phrases that acknowledge your effort to comprehend and invite further explanation. For instance, after a detailed explanation of a treatment regimen, you could say, "I'm trying to get a clear picture of how this medication works. Could you perhaps explain it using an analogy, or break down the process step-by-step for me?" Or, if a diagnosis involves complex biological processes, you might ask, "To make sure I'm following correctly, could you walk me through what's happening inside my body that leads to this diagnosis?" This approach signals that you are engaged and genuinely want to understand, rather than simply being dismissive of the information provided. It also gives the provider an opportunity to tailor their communication style to your needs, which is ultimately beneficial for your care.

Addressing anxieties and fears is another critical component of navigating difficult conversations. Sometimes, the most challenging aspects of a health condition aren't the physical symptoms themselves, but the emotional and psychological toll they take. These fears can range from the fear of pain, the fear of side effects, the fear of losing independence, to the existential fear of mortality. Openly expressing these fears can be incredibly difficult, as we may worry about being perceived as overly emotional, demanding, or even irrational. However, acknowledging and articulating these fears is a crucial step towards managing them and integrating them into a holistic care plan. Consider a scenario where a patient is recommended surgery.

Beyond the questions about the procedure itself, there might be deep-seated fears about anesthesia, recovery, or the possibility of complications. A patient might say, "I understand the surgical recommendation, and I've done my research on the procedure itself. However, I'm feeling quite anxious about the anesthesia. I've heard stories, and I'm worried about losing control or having an adverse reaction. Could we talk more about the safety protocols and what I can expect during and immediately after the anesthesia?" By vocalizing these specific worries, you open the door for your healthcare team to address them directly, providing reassurance, explaining safety measures, and perhaps even offering resources for managing pre-operative anxiety. This not only alleviates some of the patient's distress but also allows the medical team to anticipate and mitigate potential issues related to the patient's psychological state.

When the conversation turns to sensitive personal information, such as lifestyle choices, sexual health, or mental health struggles that might be linked to your physical condition, it's natural to feel a sense of trepidation. Disclosing personal details requires trust and a safe environment. The best way to foster this is to be as open and honest as you feel comfortable being, while also clearly stating your boundaries if needed. You can preface such disclosures by acknowledging the sensitivity. For example, if you suspect your stress levels are exacerbating your symptoms, you might say, "I've noticed my symptoms seem to flare up when I'm under a lot of stress at work. It's difficult for me to talk about, but I want to be upfront about this potential link. Are there ways we can explore managing both my stress and my physical symptoms?" This sets a tone of shared problem-solving. Similarly, if your symptoms have affected your intimate relationships, and you feel hesitant to discuss it, you could begin by saying, "I'm a bit embarrassed to bring this up, but I want to be thorough. My condition seems to be impacting my relationship, and I'm not sure how to navigate that. Is this something you can offer advice on, or should I speak with a specialist?" By initiating these conversations, even with a degree of hesitancy, you empower your healthcare provider to offer comprehensive support that extends beyond the purely physical.

Furthermore, difficult conversations can arise when there's a discrepancy between what you're experiencing and what the medical assessment suggests. This might happen if you feel your pain is being underestimated, or if your progress seems slower than expected. In such situations, it's crucial to approach the conversation collaboratively, focusing on your subjective experience. You can present your observations from your symptom journal as evidence. For instance, you might say, "I appreciate your assessment, but I'm still experiencing significant pain, particularly during the night. My journal shows that I've been averaging 7 out of 10 pain for the past week, which is higher than what we discussed as the target. Could we revisit my pain management strategy?" This is not an accusation, but a factual presentation of your experience. It invites a discussion about why there might be a difference between the clinical picture and your lived reality, potentially leading to adjustments in medication, therapy, or further diagnostic tests.

Navigating these conversations also involves understanding your rights as a patient and your role in shared decision-making. You have the right to understand your health information, to ask questions, and to make informed decisions about your care. When a difficult conversation is on the horizon, such as discussing treatment options with varying prognoses or significant side effects, remember that you are a partner in this process. If you are presented with a choice between two treatments, and one has a higher success rate but more severe side effects, you have the right to explore what "severe side effects" truly means for you. Ask for detailed descriptions, potential mitigation strategies, and how these side effects might impact your daily life. You can say, "I understand Treatment A has a higher success rate, but the potential side effects seem quite significant. Could you elaborate on what 'nausea' or 'fatigue' might look like in practical terms for someone undergoing this treatment? For example, would I be able to work? How would it affect my ability to care for myself?" This allows you to weigh the risks and benefits not just in abstract medical terms, but in the context of your personal life and values.

It's also important to acknowledge that sometimes, a conversation might not go as smoothly as planned, and that's okay. There might be times when you feel your concerns aren't fully heard, or that the provider is rushing through the discussion. In such instances, it's important to remain calm and assertive, rather than aggressive.

You can try reiterating your point or asking for a moment of their time. Phrases like, "I'm sorry to interrupt, but I want to make sure we've addressed my concern about X," or "Could we perhaps take a few minutes to focus specifically on the side effects, as that is my primary worry right now?" can be effective. If you still feel unheard, or if the conversation feels unproductive, it is always an option to ask if it would be possible to schedule a follow-up appointment specifically to discuss these matters further, or to request a referral to another specialist if you feel your needs are not being met. This is not about being difficult; it's about advocating for your health when the initial approach isn't sufficient.

The preparation for these difficult conversations

extends to mental preparation as well. Before an appointment, take some time to center yourself. Deep breathing exercises, mindfulness, or even writing down a few positive affirmations can help reduce anxiety and bolster your confidence. Remind yourself that your health is your priority, and you deserve clear, compassionate communication. Imagine the conversation going well, with you articulating your concerns clearly and receiving supportive, informative responses. This mental rehearsal can significantly impact your demeanor and effectiveness during the actual discussion.

For individuals managing chronic pain, the act of articulating its nature can be particularly arduous. Pain is subjective, and often, descriptions like "sharp," "dull," or "burning" are insufficient to convey the full experience. The impact of pain on daily life—the inability to sleep, the difficulty in concentrating, the social isolation—is also crucial to communicate. When discussing chronic pain, consider using a pain scale (0-10) as a starting point, but then elaborate on *what* that number represents for you. For instance, "A pain level of 8 for me means I can barely move from my bed, and I can't concentrate on anything else.

Even with medication, I'm still experiencing this level of pain most mornings." You might also want to discuss the variability of your pain. "My pain isn't constant; it fluctuates. The sharp pains are unpredictable and debilitating, and they often occur after I've been sitting for too long, even if the overall ache is manageable." Sharing these details helps the healthcare provider understand the nuances of your condition and tailor interventions more effectively. It might lead to a discussion about different pain management strategies, such as nerve blocks, physical therapy focused on specific movement patterns, or even psychological support for coping with chronic pain.

When dealing with mental health concerns that intersect with physical symptoms, such as depression impacting appetite or anxiety exacerbating digestive issues, open communication is key. It's vital to bridge the gap between the physical and the psychological. You might start by saying, "I've noticed a strong connection between my anxiety levels and my digestive problems. When I feel particularly stressed or worried, my stomach issues become much worse. I'm not sure how to address this, but I believe it's an important part of my overall health." This honest disclosure allows your healthcare team to consider integrated treatment approaches, perhaps involving both medication for the physical symptoms and referral to a therapist or counselor.

It's also important to share any over-the-counter remedies or supplements you are using, as these can sometimes interact with prescribed medications or even mask underlying symptoms. A simple statement like, "I've been taking herbal supplements for sleep and a specific vitamin for energy, alongside my prescribed medications. I wanted to mention this in case there are any interactions or if these might be affecting my symptoms," ensures a comprehensive overview of your health practices.

In conclusion, navigating difficult conversations is an art that can be learned and refined. It requires preparation, courage, clarity, and a commitment to collaborative care. By preparing your thoughts, being honest about your experiences and emotions, asking for clarification, and advocating for your needs, you transform potentially intimidating discussions into opportunities for deeper understanding and more effective treatment.

Remember, your healthcare providers are there to help you, and the more information and context you can provide, the better they can serve you.

These challenging dialogues are not obstacles; they are essential pathways to achieving your best possible health and well-being. Embrace them as integral steps in your health journey.

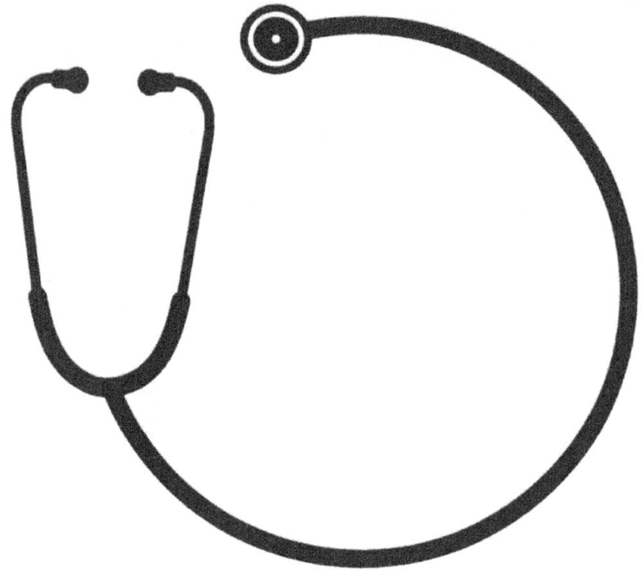

3: The Power of Bidirectional Listening

Bidirectional listening, in the realm of healthcare, transcends the conventional understanding of simply hearing words. It is not a one-way street where the patient unloads information and the provider absorbs it, or vice versa. Instead, it signifies a dynamic, reciprocal engagement where both the patient and the healthcare professional actively participate in the communication process. Unfortunately, built into the healthcare system as with the rest of our complex society is *implicit bias*—defined as unconscious attitudes, positive or negative, toward a person, group, or idea— which often leads to differential treatment based on perceived race and financial status. Implicit bias further restricts quality healthcare as a separate factor above and beyond inequities of structural racism. Imagine a skillfully orchestrated conversation, a duet rather than a monologue, where each participant is attuned to the other, seeking not just to transmit information, but to genuinely understand and be understood. This is the essence of bidirectional listening: a shared commitment to paying attention, comprehending the nuances of each other's message, and responding in a way that fosters clarity, trust, and a shared path forward. This would be in complete compliance of part of the Hippocratic Oath committing to doing what is in the best interest of the patient.

At its core, bidirectional listening is built upon the foundation of active engagement from both sides of the patient-provider relationship. For the patient, this means being present, focused, and willing to articulate their experiences, concerns, and questions with clarity and honesty, as we've explored in preceding discussions. However, the active component also extends crucially to the healthcare provider. It demands that they not only receive the patient's input but also demonstrate through their demeanor and responses that they are truly processing that information. This involves more than just nodding or jotting down notes; it means reflecting back understanding, asking clarifying questions, and signaling that the patient's narrative is being integrated into the clinical assessment. When a provider actively listens, they are not just hearing symptoms; they are hearing the lived experience behind those symptoms, the anxieties that accompany them, and the patient's personal context.

This creates a sense of validation for the patient, making them feel seen and heard, which is fundamental to building a strong therapeutic alliance.

Consider a scenario where a patient presents with a persistent cough. A provider employing unidirectional listening might focus solely on the medical characteristics of the cough: its duration, frequency, any accompanying phlegm, and potential causes like infection or asthma. While this is important, it might miss the broader impact on the patient's life. A patient experiencing a chronic cough might also be struggling with sleep deprivation, social isolation due to the embarrassment of coughing in public, or a deep-seated fear that it signifies a more serious, undiagnosed condition. Through bidirectional listening, the provider would not only inquire about the cough itself but would also create space for the patient to share these secondary concerns. The provider might ask, "How has this cough been affecting your daily life?" or "Are there any worries or fears that have come up for you because of this symptom?" By posing such questions and genuinely attending to the answers, the provider gains a more holistic understanding of the patient's situation. This allows for a more comprehensive treatment plan that might include not just medication for the cough but also strategies for managing sleep, or addressing the psychological impact of the persistent symptom. The patient, in turn, feels more understood and is more likely to adhere to the treatment plan because they see it as a collaborative effort addressing their complete well-being.

The reciprocal nature of bidirectional listening means that the onus of effective communication is shared. While patients are encouraged to be prepared and articulate, providers are equally responsible for creating an environment conducive to open dialogue. This includes managing the setting of the consultation—ensuring privacy and minimizing interruptions—as well as employing communication techniques that encourage patient participation. Using open-ended questions, paraphrasing what the patient has said to confirm understanding, and allowing for moments of silence where the patient can gather their thoughts are all hallmarks of bidirectional listening from the provider's end. It's about fostering a partnership where the patient feels empowered to contribute actively to their own care, knowing that their input is valued and will shape the decisions made.

Furthermore, bidirectional listening plays a critical role in accurate diagnosis. Listening is transformational—for students, for teachers, and for leaders. It is a skill that must be taught, nurtured, and practiced at every level of our educational system to include medical schools if we are going to commit to the health of all. Often, subtle cues or seemingly minor details shared by a patient can be the key to unlocking a complex medical puzzle. Without a listening style that encourages the patient to elaborate and a provider who is receptive to these nuances, vital diagnostic information can be overlooked. Imagine a patient describing a rash. Unidirectional listening might focus on the visual appearance of the rash: its color, texture, and location. Bidirectional listening, however, would prompt the provider to ask about the onset, any associated symptoms like itching or burning, what makes it better or worse, and importantly, any recent changes in the patient's environment, diet, or lifestyle that might be relevant. Perhaps the patient mentions, almost as an afterthought, that the rash appeared after starting a new laundry detergent or spending time gardening in a particular area. These seemingly tangential pieces of information, when actively listened to and explored, can be crucial in identifying the root cause of the rash, whether it's an allergic reaction, an infection, or something else entirely. This level of detail and context is only uncovered when the listening is a two-way street, where both parties are actively engaged in uncovering the full picture.

The concept also extends to the provider's explanation of diagnoses and treatment plans. Bidirectional listening means that once the provider has explained something, they must then actively listen to the patient's response to gauge their understanding and address any lingering questions or concerns. This might involve observing the patient's body language, noting any signs of confusion or apprehension, and then prompting them to express any doubts. This type of skill is not just instinctive for a provider but must be taught as a skill to be an effective provider in this new model of healthcare which needs to become more inclusive of all. A provider might say, "I've explained the rationale for this treatment and the expected outcomes. Does that make sense to you? Are there any parts that are unclear, or any aspects you'd like me to elaborate on further?" This isn't just a perfunctory question; it's an invitation for the patient to engage with the information, to process it, and to voice any disconnects between the provider's explanation and their own comprehension. When the patient responds with specific questions, such as "You mentioned 'renal clearance,' could you explain what that means in practical terms for my kidney function?" or "What are the specific signs I should watch out for that indicate the medication isn't working as expected?", they are actively participating in the listening process, ensuring they receive information tailored to their understanding. This mutual feedback loop is what transforms information transfer into genuine understanding and shared decision-making.

The effectiveness of bidirectional listening is also deeply intertwined with the development of trust and rapport between patient and provider. When patients feel that their healthcare providers are genuinely listening to them, taking their concerns seriously, and valuing their input, a strong bond of trust is forged. This trust is not merely a pleasant byproduct of good communication; it is foundational to effective healthcare. A trusting patient is more likely to be open about sensitive information, to adhere to treatment recommendations, and to feel comfortable seeking help when new issues arise. Conversely, a patient who feels unheard or dismissed by their provider may become disengaged, less likely to seek medical attention when needed, and more prone to mistrust medical advice. Bidirectional listening actively cultivates this trust by demonstrating respect for the patient as an individual with unique experiences and perspectives.

Consider the psychological aspect of illness. Many conditions carry significant emotional weight, and patients often need to express their fears, anxieties, or frustrations to their providers. A provider who engages in bidirectional listening creates a safe space for these emotions to be shared. For instance, a patient recently diagnosed with a chronic illness might express feelings of hopelessness or anger. A provider employing unidirectional listening might focus on the objective medical management of the illness, perhaps offering statistics or treatment protocols.

However, a provider practicing bidirectional listening would acknowledge these emotional expressions. They might say, "It sounds like you're feeling overwhelmed by this diagnosis, and that's completely understandable. Many people feel a range of emotions when facing a new health challenge. Would you like to talk more about how this is affecting you emotionally, or perhaps discuss resources that could help you cope with these feelings?" This open acknowledgment and invitation to discuss emotional well-being demonstrates that the provider values the patient's holistic health, encompassing both physical and psychological aspects. This fosters a sense of partnership and shared responsibility for managing the illness, rather than a purely clinical, detached approach.

The implementation of bidirectional listening also requires an awareness of potential communication barriers, and a willingness from both parties to overcome them.

These barriers can range from language differences

and cultural misunderstandings to differing levels of health literacy and the inherent power imbalance in the patient-provider relationship. Bidirectional listening actively seeks to mitigate these barriers. For a provider, this might involve using plain language, employing visual aids, or utilizing interpreter services when necessary. For a patient, it means being prepared to ask for clarification if something is not understood, or to express concerns about cultural sensitivities. When these efforts are made mutually, it signifies a shared commitment to bridging any gaps in understanding, reinforcing the collaborative nature of the healthcare encounter. For example, if a provider uses a medical term that the patient doesn't understand, a bidirectional listening approach would involve the patient saying, "I'm sorry, I'm not familiar with that term. Could you explain it in simpler language?" And the provider, in turn, would readily provide a more accessible explanation, perhaps using an analogy, without making the patient feel inadequate for not knowing the term.

The commitment to bidirectional listening extends beyond a single consultation; it is an ongoing process that underpins the entire patient-provider relationship. It means that at every touchpoint, from initial diagnosis to ongoing management and treatment adjustments, the principles of active engagement, mutual understanding, and respectful dialogue are upheld. When treatment plans need to be modified, or when a patient experiences unexpected side effects, bidirectional listening ensures that the patient's feedback is actively sought and considered. For instance, if a patient reports that a medication is causing significant side effects, a provider practicing bidirectional listening would not dismiss these reports but would actively explore them. They would ask detailed questions about the nature, timing, and severity of the side effects, and then collaboratively discuss potential solutions, such as adjusting the dosage, switching to a different medication, or managing the side effects themselves. This iterative process of communication, listening, and adjustment is vital for optimizing treatment outcomes and ensuring patient satisfaction and safety. It demonstrates a provider's responsiveness to the patient's evolving needs and experiences, solidifying the foundation of trust and partnership.

In essence, bidirectional listening transforms the healthcare interaction from a clinical transaction into a therapeutic partnership. It elevates the patient from a passive recipient of care to an active collaborator, empowered to contribute their unique insights and experiences. Simultaneously, it encourages healthcare providers to move beyond a purely diagnostic and prescriptive role to become engaged listeners, empathetic communicators, and genuine partners in the patient's health journey. This mutual engagement fosters a more effective, personalized, and ultimately more human approach to healthcare, where the shared goal of achieving optimal health and well-being is pursued through open communication and mutual understanding. It is this dynamic, reciprocal exchange that forms the bedrock of truly patient-centered care.

The commitment to bidirectional listening is a shared responsibility, and while the healthcare provider plays a crucial role in fostering an environment of open communication, the patient's active participation as a listener is equally vital. This section delves into the patient's role in this crucial dialogue, equipping you with the tools and mindset to become a more effective listener during your healthcare interactions. It's not merely about being present in the room; it's about being mentally and emotionally engaged, ready to receive, process, and respond to the information being shared. Think of it as a collaborative effort to decipher a complex set of instructions that directly impact your well-being. When you actively listen, you not only gain a deeper understanding of your health condition and treatment plan but also contribute significantly to the accuracy of the information being exchanged, ensuring that the care you receive is truly tailored to your needs.

One of the foundational elements of active listening for patients is the ability to concentrate. In today's world, distractions are ubiquitous. Your mind might wander to upcoming appointments, work deadlines, or personal concerns, especially when you are feeling unwell or anxious. To combat this, consciously make an effort to be present in the moment. This might involve putting your phone away, consciously setting aside intrusive thoughts, and directing your full attention to the healthcare provider. A simple technique is to maintain eye contact, not in an aggressive way, but as a signal that you are engaged and receptive. When the provider is speaking, try to clear your mental slate and focus on their words, their tone of voice, and any visual aids they might be using. This focused attention allows you to absorb the information more effectively, reducing the likelihood of missing critical details. Imagine the difference between trying to read a book in a noisy, bustling cafe versus in a quiet library; the latter allows for much deeper comprehension. Similarly, a focused mind allows for a deeper understanding of medical information.

Processing the information you receive is the next critical step. It's not enough to just hear the words; you need to make sense of them. This involves mentally organizing the information, connecting it to what you already know about your health, and identifying any points of confusion. Healthcare providers often impart a significant amount of technical or complex information during a consultation. Your role as an active listener is to engage with this information, to think about what it means for you, and to identify areas where you might need further clarification. This might involve mentally summarizing what the provider has said, or trying to anticipate what they might say next based on the context. For instance, if a doctor is explaining a new medication, you might be processing details about its purpose, how it works, its dosage, potential side effects, and how it fits into your overall treatment plan. This internal processing helps solidify the information and prepares you to ask relevant questions.

Asking clarifying questions is an indispensable part of being an active listener. It signals to the provider that you are engaged and that you are taking your health seriously. It also serves as a crucial mechanism for ensuring accuracy and understanding. If something is unclear, ambiguous, or if you simply want more detail, do not hesitate to ask. This is not a sign of weakness or ignorance; it is a sign of responsible self-advocacy. For example, if a provider mentions a specific medical term that you are unfamiliar with, such as "hypertension" or "metabolism," it is perfectly acceptable to ask, "Could you please explain what 'hypertension' means in relation to my blood pressure?" or "When you talk about my metabolism, what specific aspects are we discussing?" These questions are vital for demystifying medical jargon and ensuring that you have a clear grasp of your condition and treatment. Similarly, if the rationale behind a particular treatment or diagnostic test is not immediately apparent, asking for an explanation can foster a better understanding of the medical process. For instance, you might ask, "I understand you want me to have this blood test, but could you explain why this particular test is important for my diagnosis?"

A powerful technique for confirming your understanding is paraphrasing. This involves restating what the provider has said in your own words. It serves as a double-check, ensuring that you have interpreted the information correctly and giving the provider an opportunity to correct any misunderstandings. For example, after a doctor explains a treatment plan, you might say, "So, if I understand correctly, you're recommending that I take this medication twice a day, and I should expect to see some improvement in my symptoms within two weeks. Is that right?" This not only confirms your comprehension but also reinforces the information in your own mind. The provider's affirmation or gentle correction of your paraphrase provides immediate feedback, bridging any gaps in communication before they can become significant issues. This collaborative approach to confirming understanding builds confidence and ensures that both parties are on the same page.

Avoiding distractions is paramount to effective listening. This extends beyond just your phone; it also includes internal distractions such as anxiety or preoccupation with your symptoms. When you are in a healthcare setting, try to focus on the interaction at hand. If you are feeling overwhelmed by anxiety, it is perfectly acceptable to acknowledge this to your provider. You might say, "I'm feeling a bit anxious about all this information, so I might ask you to repeat a few things." A good provider will understand and appreciate your honesty. Furthermore, be mindful of external distractions in the room. If there are interruptions, or if you are struggling to hear over background noise, it is appropriate to politely address this. You might say, "Excuse me, I'm having a little trouble hearing. Could we perhaps speak a bit louder, or is there a quieter space we could move to?" These are not demands, but rather requests aimed at facilitating clear communication for your benefit.

Another aspect of active listening is being prepared to provide relevant information concisely. While the focus here is on listening, effective bidirectional communication requires both speaking and listening well. When the provider asks questions, listen carefully to what they are asking and provide clear, focused answers. Avoid rambling or going off on tangents that might distract from the core issue. For example, if asked about your pain, try to describe its location, intensity, quality (e.g., sharp, dull, throbbing), and what makes it better or worse, rather than launching into a long narrative about unrelated life events. This preparation helps ensure that the information exchange is efficient and productive, allowing more time for the provider to explain and for you to listen and understand. Before your appointment, it can be incredibly helpful to jot down your symptoms, any questions you have, and any information you think the provider might need. This preparation allows you to listen more effectively, as you have already organized your own thoughts and concerns.

It's also important to be aware of your own non-verbal cues as a listener. Your body language can communicate your level of engagement. Sitting up, facing the provider, and nodding occasionally can signal that you are attentive. Conversely, looking away frequently, fidgeting excessively, or appearing disengaged can inadvertently communicate a lack of interest, even if that is not your intention. While you are not expected to be a therapist, being mindful of your presence can enhance the communicative flow. This doesn't mean you need to force a smile or pretend everything is fine if it isn't, but rather to present yourself as someone who is open to receiving information and engaging in the dialogue about your health.

Furthermore, active listening involves being receptive to information that may be difficult to hear. This could include diagnoses that are serious, treatment side effects that are unpleasant, or lifestyle changes that require significant adjustments. While it's natural to feel disappointment, fear, or even denial in such situations, an active listener strives to process this information as objectively as possible. This doesn't mean suppressing your emotions, but rather acknowledging them and then making a conscious effort to understand the clinical implications. For example, if a provider explains that a certain medication has a known side effect that you are concerned about, an active listener would process this information and then formulate questions focused on understanding the risk-benefit ratio, or strategies to manage that specific side effect, rather than simply dismissing the medication outright due to the mention of a side effect. This balanced approach is key to making informed decisions about your care.

The patient's role in active listening also extends to observing the provider's non-verbal communication. While you are focused on their words, pay attention to their tone of voice, their facial expressions, and their overall demeanor. These can offer additional layers of information. A provider who speaks with empathy and warmth, for instance, might be conveying a deeper level of understanding or concern than one who speaks in a more detached manner. Similarly, if a provider seems rushed or distracted, it might signal that you need to be more direct with your questions or ask if it's a good time to discuss your concerns in more depth. This awareness of the provider's non-verbal cues allows you to better interpret the overall communication dynamic.

Consider the common scenario of receiving a prescription. A healthcare provider might explain the dosage, frequency, and the intended effect of the medication. An active listener patient wouldn't just nod and take the paper. They would process this information: "So, it's one pill, twice a day, with food, to help lower my blood pressure. What happens if I miss a dose? Are there any common side effects I should watch out for that are different from what was mentioned? How long will I need to take this medication?" Asking these follow-up questions demonstrates active listening and a commitment to understanding the full scope of the treatment. It also provides the provider with valuable feedback about what aspects of the information might need further emphasis or clarification. This proactive engagement can prevent misunderstandings about medication adherence, which is a significant factor in treatment success.

The practice of active listening by patients is also

crucial for identifying potential concerns or errors early on. If a provider's explanation seems contradictory, or if the information they provide doesn't align with your personal experience or other information you may have gathered (from reputable sources, of course), speaking up is essential. For example, if you have been managing a particular symptom in a certain way that has been effective for you, and the provider suggests a completely different approach without acknowledging your current method, it might be worth gently inquiring. You could say, "I've been using X method to manage this, and it's been helpful. Could you explain how this new approach might be better or different for my situation?" This kind of dialogue, born from active listening and informed by your lived experience, can lead to more nuanced and effective care plans.

Ultimately, becoming an active listener patient is about adopting a mindset of partnership and shared responsibility in your healthcare journey. It's about recognizing that your active participation in the communication process is as important as the provider's. By concentrating on what is being said, processing the information, asking clarifying questions, paraphrasing to confirm understanding, and avoiding distractions, you empower yourself to be a more informed and engaged participant in your own care. This not only leads to a better understanding of your health and treatment but also strengthens the therapeutic alliance with your healthcare provider, paving the way for more effective, personalized, and positive health outcomes. It transforms the clinical encounter from a one-sided delivery of information into a dynamic, collaborative dialogue focused on your well-being.

When you are a patient navigating the complexities of healthcare, the exchange of information with your provider is paramount. As we've explored the patient's role in this vital dialogue, it's equally important to equip you with the ability to recognize when the provider is truly engaging in bidirectional listening. This is not about judging their medical expertise, but rather about understanding the quality of the communication dynamic. By observing specific behaviors, you can gain confidence that your voice is being heard, understood, and valued, which in turn can significantly enhance your overall experience and the effectiveness of your care. Recognizing these signs allows you to feel more assured that your concerns are not just being processed, but are genuinely being considered as part of your treatment journey.

One of the most immediate and universally recognized indicators of active listening is **sustained eye contact**. When a provider maintains appropriate eye contact while you are speaking, it signals that their attention is directed towards you. This isn't about an intense, unbroken stare, which can feel unnerving, but rather a comfortable and natural engagement with your gaze. It's a non-verbal cue that communicates presence and focus. Think of it as a silent acknowledgment that you are the center of their attention at that moment, that they are present with you in the conversation.

This can be particularly reassuring when you are discussing sensitive or difficult health issues, where feeling seen and acknowledged can make a significant difference in your comfort level and willingness to share openly. When a provider's eyes are frequently darting to the computer screen, the clock, or the door, it can create a sense of being rushed or unimportant, even if that's not their intention. Therefore, noticing consistent, natural eye contact is a positive sign that your provider is tuned in.

Beyond eye contact, pay attention to **attentive body language**. This includes subtle yet significant cues such as nodding in response to what you are saying, leaning slightly forward, or orienting their body towards you. These actions convey engagement and an openness to receive your message. A provider who is actively listening will often mirror a sense of calm and receptiveness through their posture. Imagine a provider who remains seated with their arms crossed, or who appears physically withdrawn; these stances can inadvertently create a barrier to communication. Conversely, a provider who appears relaxed yet attentive, with open posture and a calm demeanor, is more likely to be processing your words and emotions effectively. These non-verbal affirmations, such as a gentle nod or a slight lean, provide unspoken validation that you are being heard and understood, fostering a more comfortable and productive interaction.

A crucial sign of active listening is the provider's **tendency to ask relevant follow-up questions**. This demonstrates that they are not just passively receiving information but are actively processing it, seeking clarification, and delving deeper into your concerns. For example, if you mention a particular symptom, an actively listening provider might ask, "Can you describe that pain in more detail? For instance, is it sharp, dull, or throbbing?" or "When did you first notice this symptom appearing?" These types of questions indicate that they are engaged with the specifics of your experience and are trying to build a comprehensive picture of your health. It's the difference between a provider who simply records your initial statement and one who probes further to gain a richer understanding. Asking for elaboration on a symptom, its onset, duration, or impact on your daily life are all hallmarks of a provider who is truly listening and trying to connect the dots. This also helps the patient to organize their own thoughts and provide more precise information.

Furthermore, actively listening providers will often **summarize or paraphrase** what you have said. This technique is a powerful way for them to confirm their understanding and ensure that they have accurately interpreted your concerns. You might hear a provider say something like, "So, if I'm understanding correctly, you've been experiencing headaches primarily in the afternoon, and they seem to be exacerbated by screen time. Is that right?" This not only verifies that they've grasped the key points but also gives you an opportunity to correct any misunderstandings. This shared understanding is a bedrock of effective care, preventing misinterpretations that could lead to incorrect diagnoses or treatment plans. When a provider can accurately restate your main concerns, it provides immense reassurance that they are not just hearing the words, but comprehending the meaning and significance behind them. It's a collaborative effort to ensure alignment.

Another valuable indicator is the provider's **response to your questions**. An actively listening provider will not only answer your questions but will do so in a way that is clear, understandable, and addresses the core of your inquiry. They will avoid dismissiveness or impatience and will take the time to explain complex medical terms or concepts. If you ask a question and the provider offers a vague or evasive answer, or if they seem annoyed by your questions, it might suggest that they are not fully engaged in the listening process. Conversely, a provider who patiently breaks down a treatment plan, explains potential side effects, or clarifies the purpose of a diagnostic test, is demonstrating that they value your understanding and are committed to open communication. For instance, if you ask about medication side effects, a good listener will not only list them but might also explain their likelihood, severity, and management strategies, showing they have considered your potential concerns.

Minimizing distractions during your conversation is also a strong signal of a provider's attentiveness. While it's understood that healthcare professionals often have demanding schedules and may need to check electronic health records, an actively listening provider will strive to minimize interruptions and maintain focus on you. If they need to consult the electronic record, they might say, "I just need to check your chart for a moment to confirm some information," rather than silently typing while you're talking. They will also be mindful of ambient noise or other distractions and may take steps to mitigate them, such as closing a door or asking a colleague to wait. This conscious effort to create a focused environment underscores their commitment to giving you their undivided attention. When a provider consistently puts their phone away, closes their computer screen momentarily to engage with you, or ensures a degree of privacy, it communicates respect for your time and your concerns.

Observe how the provider **integrates your input into their assessment**. An actively listening provider will weave the information you provide into their diagnostic process. They won't just gather a list of symptoms; they will connect those symptoms to your medical history, your lifestyle, and the physical examination findings. This integration shows that your perspective is actively being used to inform their professional judgment. For example, if you mention that a particular activity consistently triggers your symptoms, and the provider then asks specific questions about that activity and its relationship to your physical presentation, it signifies that your personal experience is being taken seriously and utilized in the diagnostic reasoning. This is more than just data collection;

it's a synthesis of your narrative with their medical knowledge.

Consider the **quality and clarity of their explanations**. When a provider explains a diagnosis, a treatment plan, or a next step, the clarity and comprehensibility of that explanation are directly related to how well they have listened and understood your situation. If their explanations are clear, logical, and directly address the issues you've raised, it's a strong indication of attentive listening. Conversely, if explanations are confusing, contradictory, or seem disconnected from what you've communicated, it may signal that there's a disconnect in the listening process. For example, if you've expressed significant concern about a particular side effect, and the provider's explanation of how to manage it is thorough and reassuring, it shows they've not only heard your concern but have also processed its significance for you.

It is also important to acknowledge that **emotional attunement** can be a subtle but powerful indicator of active listening. While providers are expected to maintain professional boundaries, an ability to show empathy and acknowledge your emotional state can be a sign that they are listening on a deeper level. This might manifest as a provider saying, "I understand this must be a difficult diagnosis to hear," or "It's perfectly normal to feel worried about this," accompanied by a tone of voice and facial expression that convey genuine concern. This emotional connection, when present, suggests that the provider is not just processing the medical facts but also recognizing the human impact of your health condition. It builds trust and makes the patient feel more like a partner in their care, rather than just a case to be managed.

When a provider reflects on your past experiences or stated preferences, it's another sign of attentive listening. For instance, if you mention that you prefer not to take certain types of medications due to past adverse reactions or personal beliefs, and the provider remembers this and incorporates it into their recommendations, it shows they are listening and remembering details that are important to you. This personalized approach to care is a direct result of the provider's commitment to truly hearing and valuing the patient's input. It's about building a shared understanding of what effective and acceptable care looks like *for you*, based on what you have shared.

Finally, consider the **provider's overall demeanor and approachability**. While not a direct listening behavior, a provider who creates an environment where you feel comfortable speaking up, asking questions, and even disagreeing respectfully is one who is likely practicing good listening skills. If you feel you can interrupt politely to ask for clarification without causing offense, or if you feel encouraged to share any anxieties you might have, these are all signs of a positive communication dynamic. A provider who is perceived as approachable and open is often one who is also a good listener, as these qualities tend to go hand-in-hand. This overarching feeling of trust and respect in the patient-provider relationship is often built on a foundation of effective, bidirectional listening. By consciously observing these cues, you can gain a clearer understanding of how well your healthcare provider is engaging with you, fostering a more empowered and collaborative healthcare experience.

Bridging the communication gap is a crucial skill for any patient seeking to optimize their healthcare experience and outcomes. While identifying a good listener is important, actively participating in ensuring clarity and understanding is equally vital. Misunderstandings in healthcare can range from minor inconveniences to serious errors, impacting treatment efficacy, patient safety, and overall satisfaction.

Therefore, proactively addressing potential misinterpretations and ensuring alignment between patient and provider is not just beneficial; it's a fundamental aspect of collaborative care. This subsection will delve into practical strategies you can employ to bridge any communication gaps that may arise, fostering a more robust and accurate exchange of information.

One of the most effective strategies for bridging communication gaps is the practice of **summarizing key points** after a discussion. This involves rephrasing the most important information exchanged in your own words. For instance, after discussing a new medication, you might say, "So, to make sure I've understood correctly, I should take this pill twice a day, with food, and it might cause some drowsiness. Is that right?" This simple act serves multiple purposes. Firstly, it allows the provider to confirm whether their message was received as intended. If there's a discrepancy, they can immediately clarify. Secondly, it reinforces the information in your own mind, making it easier to recall and follow later. This might be particularly helpful when dealing with complex treatment regimens or when you are feeling overwhelmed by a diagnosis. Imagine you've just received instructions for a new diagnostic test involving dietary restrictions and specific timing for medication. A quick summary like, "So, I need to fast for 12 hours before the test, and I should bring my current list of medications with me when I come in," allows the provider to verify that you've grasped the essential preparations. This simple act transforms passive reception into active engagement with the information, solidifying your understanding and the provider's confidence in your comprehension. It's a proactive measure that significantly reduces the likelihood of errors stemming from misremembered or misunderstood instructions.

Beyond summarizing, **confirming your understanding of instructions** is paramount, especially when it comes to actions you need to take. This involves not just repeating what was said, but articulating your planned actions based on those instructions. For example, if a provider tells you to monitor your blood pressure and call if it exceeds a certain number, you could respond by saying, "I will check my blood pressure every morning and evening. If it reads 140 over 90 or higher, I will call the office to report it." This level of detail demonstrates a deeper engagement with the instructions and provides the provider with concrete evidence that you know what to do and when. Consider a scenario where a physical therapist provides exercises for rehabilitation. Instead of just nodding, you might say, "Okay, so I'll do these 10 repetitions of the leg raises three times a day, making sure to hold the stretch for 30 seconds each time. I'll do them before breakfast, after lunch, and before dinner." This detailed confirmation assures the therapist that you understand the frequency, duration, and form of the exercises, minimizing the risk of ineffective or even harmful execution. This proactive confirmation empowers you by ensuring you are clear on your responsibilities in your care plan and gives the provider peace of mind that their instructions are being accurately translated into action. It's about ensuring that the care plan is not just communicated, but also internalized and executable by you, the patient.

There are times when, despite best efforts, you might feel that information is still unclear or that you may have missed something. In these instances, **politely seeking repetition or clarification** is not a sign of weakness or lack of intelligence, but a testament to your commitment to accurate care. You can phrase this by saying, "I'm sorry, could you please repeat that last instruction?" or "I want to make sure I understand this correctly. Could you explain the difference between 'acute' and 'chronic' pain again?" It is important to do this in a way that is respectful of the provider's time and expertise. Phrases like "I apologize for asking again, but..." or "To be absolutely sure..." can soften the request. Providers who are truly engaged listeners will appreciate your desire for clarity and will be happy to re-explain.

Imagine you are discussing the side effects of a medication, and the provider mentions a particular reaction, but you didn't quite catch the name or its significance. Instead of letting it pass, you could say,

"Excuse me, I didn't quite catch the name of that rare side effect you mentioned. Could you say it again, and perhaps explain what symptoms I should watch for?" This shows that you are paying attention and are invested in understanding potential risks. Similarly, if you are receiving instructions for a complex procedure, and a step seems ambiguous, asking for a re-explanation of that specific step is crucial. For example, "I'm still a little unclear about the preparation for the colonoscopy - specifically, when I should stop eating solid foods. Could you go over that part one more time?" This ensures that you are not acting on incomplete or potentially flawed understanding. When a provider uses jargon, or when the pace of information delivery is rapid, seeking clarification becomes even more critical. A phrase like, "I'm not familiar with that medical term. Could you tell me what that means in simpler terms?" is perfectly acceptable and encouraged. This open communication loop ensures that no detail is overlooked and that your care is based on a solid foundation of shared understanding.

Furthermore, it's beneficial to **articulate any assumptions you might be making**. Sometimes, we might interpret information based on our own experiences or prior knowledge, which might not align with the provider's intent. For example, if a provider says, "We need to monitor your vital signs closely," you might assume this means hourly checks. You could then clarify by saying, "When you say 'closely,' does that mean checking my temperature and pulse every hour, or is there a different frequency you have in mind?" This helps to uncover potential divergences in understanding before they lead to errors. Consider a situation where a doctor prescribes a particular type of bandage for a wound. You might assume it's a waterproof bandage, especially if you have an active lifestyle. Clarifying this by asking, "Is this bandage suitable for showering, or should I replace it with a waterproof one before I bathe?" can prevent the wound from becoming compromised. By verbalizing your assumptions, you create an opportunity for the provider to correct them and provide accurate guidance, ensuring that your actions align with the medical recommendations. This proactive approach to assumption-checking is a powerful tool in preventing the subtle miscommunications that can have significant downstream effects on your health.

When it comes to instructions that involve **specific timelines or sequences**, it's essential to confirm these details explicitly. For instance, if you're told to take medication before or after a meal, or to perform a certain action within a particular timeframe, restating this ensures accuracy. You might say, "Just to be clear, I should take this antibiotic capsule an hour before eating, and then the pain reliever with my meal?" or "So, I need to apply the cream to the affected area twice a day, once in the morning after I get up, and again before I go to bed?" This precision is critical for treatments that depend on the timing of administration, absorption, or interaction with other bodily processes. Think about instructions for managing a chronic condition like diabetes, which often involves a precise sequence of events like blood sugar monitoring, insulin injection, and meal consumption. Confirming the order, "So, first I check my blood sugar, then I administer the insulin if it's needed, and then I have my breakfast within 30 minutes?" ensures that the critical steps are performed in the correct order for effective blood sugar control. This meticulous attention to detail in timing and sequencing is a cornerstone of safe and effective self-management of health conditions.

Another aspect of bridging communication gaps involves **understanding the 'why' behind instructions**. When you comprehend the rationale for a particular recommendation, it not only increases your adherence but also helps you to better troubleshoot if unexpected issues arise. Instead of just accepting an instruction, consider asking, "Could you explain why it's important for me to avoid X while I'm taking this medication?" or "What is the benefit of doing this particular exercise?" For example, if a doctor advises a low-sodium diet, asking, "Why is reducing sodium so important for my condition?" might lead to an explanation about its impact on blood pressure and fluid retention, which can deepen your understanding and motivation. Similarly, if a therapist recommends a specific range of motion for a joint, inquiring about the physiological reason behind it can be enlightening. "Why is it important to not push beyond this point during the stretch?" might elicit an explanation about preventing scar tissue formation or re-injury. When providers take the time to explain the underlying principles, it transforms instructions from arbitrary rules into actionable knowledge, empowering you to take a more active and informed role in your health. This deeper understanding also equips you to recognize when your body's response might be deviating from the expected outcomes, prompting you to seek further guidance sooner.

Furthermore, **documenting your understanding** can be an invaluable tool. While not a direct communication *during* the appointment, it's a vital step in solidifying what was discussed and ensuring you can refer back to it later. This could involve jotting down notes during the visit, or immediately afterward, summarizing the key points, instructions, and follow-up actions. Some patients find it helpful to use a dedicated notebook or a smartphone app for this purpose. For instance, after an appointment, you might write down: "Dr. Smith: Diagnosis - [condition]. Treatment - [medication name], take 1 tablet twice daily with food. Next steps - Blood test next week, schedule follow-up in 3 weeks. Key concerns addressed - [list]." This personal record serves as a reliable reference, especially if you are managing multiple health conditions or seeing several specialists. It can also be a useful resource if you need to consult with another healthcare professional or if you experience changes in your symptoms and want to recall previous advice. Imagine being discharged from the hospital after surgery. The instructions for wound care, medication, and activity levels can be extensive. Having a written summary of these instructions, perhaps even taken down by a family member or friend, can prevent confusion and ensure proper recovery.

This self-generated documentation acts as a personal quality assurance check on the communication you received, ensuring that critical details are not lost in the busy flow of healthcare.

When discussing potential **risks and benefits** of treatments or procedures, ensure you have a clear grasp of both. This involves not just understanding what the benefits are, but also the likelihood and severity of potential risks. If a provider lists risks without context, don't hesitate to ask for clarification. For example, if they mention a risk of infection, you could ask, "What is the approximate percentage of patients who experience this side effect?" or "What are the specific signs and symptoms of infection I should be looking out for?" This pursuit of clarity helps you make truly informed decisions. Consider a scenario where a surgical procedure is recommended. The surgeon might list potential complications like bleeding or nerve damage. A patient might then ask, "What is the success rate of this surgery?" or "How likely is it that I would experience significant bleeding, and what measures are in place to manage it if it occurs?" This level of inquiry allows for a more balanced understanding of the trade-offs involved and enables you to ask pertinent questions that lead to a more informed consent process. It's about moving beyond a superficial understanding of risks and benefits to a nuanced appreciation of what they mean for your individual situation.

It is also crucial to address **any perceived inconsistencies** in the information provided. If you notice that information from one provider seems to contradict advice from another, or even information from the same provider at different times, it's important to raise this. Gently pointing out the discrepancy can help resolve confusion. You might say, "I remember you mentioning last time that I should avoid X, but today you recommended Y. Could you help me understand the change or if I've misunderstood something?" For instance, if you are seeing both a cardiologist and a primary care physician, and their recommendations regarding a particular medication or lifestyle change differ, it's essential to bring this to their attention, perhaps by sharing notes from one appointment with the other, or by asking for their inter-physician consultation. This cross-referencing ensures that your care is integrated and consistent. Imagine you've received conflicting advice on managing your blood sugar from your endocrinologist and a nutritionist. Bringing both sets of advice to one of them, or even to a combined consultation if possible, allows for a consolidated and clear plan. This proactive approach to resolving inconsistencies prevents you from navigating potentially conflicting advice and ensures that your treatment plan is cohesive and well-coordinated.

Finally, remember that **building a relationship of trust and open communication** with your healthcare providers is an ongoing process. Each interaction is an opportunity to refine your communication skills and to strengthen the partnership you have with your care team. By employing these strategies – summarizing, confirming, seeking clarification, understanding the 'why', documenting, and addressing inconsistencies - you actively participate in bridging any communication gaps. This not only enhances your understanding and adherence to your treatment plan but also fosters a more collaborative and effective healthcare experience, ultimately leading to better health outcomes. It is through this active and engaged approach that you can truly harness the power of bidirectional listening, ensuring your voice is not only heard but also accurately understood and acted upon. This proactive engagement transforms you from a passive recipient of care into an empowered partner, co-creating your health journey with your providers.

When listening falls short, and you find yourself in a healthcare setting where your concerns feel unheard or misunderstood, it's easy to feel frustrated, dismissed, or even anxious. This is a common, albeit disheartening, experience for many patients. The goal of bidirectional listening is to create a harmonious exchange of information, but like any human interaction, it's not always perfect. When you sense that the channel of communication is breaking down, it's crucial to have a toolkit of strategies to help steer the conversation back on course. This isn't about assigning blame; it's about proactively ensuring your health needs are met with the clarity and attention they deserve.

The first step in addressing a perceived listening deficit is to politely but firmly **reiterate your concern**. Often, a simple restatement can reset the conversation. Rather than assuming the provider is intentionally disregarding your point, consider that they might be focused on a different aspect of your condition, or perhaps they simply missed the nuance of what you were trying to convey. You could try saying, "I appreciate you explaining X, but I'm still concerned about Y. Could we revisit that for a moment?" or "I feel like we might have slightly different understandings about my symptoms. To clarify, what I'm experiencing is [describe again] and it's making me worried about [explain impact]." For instance, imagine you've discussed a new pain medication, and the doctor has explained its benefits. However, you haven't managed to convey the severity of the side effect - say, severe nausea - that is preventing you from taking it. Instead of accepting their reassurances about common side effects, you might say, "I understand that nausea can be a side effect, but for me, it's been so intense that I haven't been able to keep the medication down at all. I'm worried about this and need to find a different solution." This direct, yet polite, restatement brings the focus back to your specific experience and the impact it's having. Another scenario could be discussing a diagnostic test. The provider might explain the procedure itself, but you're concerned about the recovery period and how it will affect your ability to care for your young children. You might then interject, "Thank you for explaining the steps of the MRI. My main concern right now, however, is how long the recovery will take and if I'll be able to lift my children shortly after the procedure. Could we discuss that aspect?" By framing it as a need for clarification and expressing your worry, you invite the provider to acknowledge and address the part of your concern that may have been overlooked. This approach demonstrates that you are engaged in the process and are seeking a comprehensive understanding of your care plan.

When reiterating doesn't seem to achieve the

desired clarity, it's time to **ask specific, targeted questions** that pinpoint the area of misunderstanding. Broad statements can be easily misinterpreted, but focused inquiries require a more direct response. If you feel your question about a particular symptom has been glossed over, instead of saying "You're not listening to me about my pain," try asking, "When I mentioned the sharp, shooting pain in my leg, what potential causes were you considering for that specific type of pain?" or "Regarding the medication dosage, could you clarify the exact reasoning for the increase from 5mg to 10mg, given my current blood pressure readings?" This forces the provider to address the specifics of your query. Consider a situation where you've been discussing a treatment plan for a chronic condition, and you feel the lifestyle modifications proposed are too generic. You might ask, "You've suggested I should reduce my sugar intake. Given my specific diagnosis of [condition], are there particular types of sugars I should focus on avoiding, or are there any fruits that would be particularly beneficial for me to include?" This narrows the scope of the discussion and prompts a more personalized response. Another example could be after receiving instructions for a wound dressing change. If you feel the instructions for hygiene were vague, you might ask, "What is the recommended antiseptic solution for cleaning the wound before applying the new dressing, and should I be using sterile gloves or just washing my hands thoroughly?" Such precise questions demonstrate that you are paying attention and are seeking concrete, actionable guidance. They create an opening for the provider to offer more detailed explanations and address the specifics of your situation, rather than relying on general advice.

If you find that verbal communication is proving challenging, **explore alternative communication methods**. Not all providers are equally adept at all forms of communication, and sometimes a shift in modality can be highly effective. If you are feeling rushed or unable to articulate your thoughts clearly in real-time, consider writing down your key concerns and questions beforehand and presenting them. You could say, "I've written down a few points I wanted to make sure we cover today.

Would it be alright if I read them out or handed you

this list?" This ensures that your most important points are not forgotten. For instance, if you're dealing with a complex medical history or multiple issues, a written list can act as a prompt for both you and the provider, ensuring all critical topics are addressed. Imagine you're seeing a specialist for a rare condition, and you want to be sure you cover all aspects of your treatment plan. Preparing a list of questions about medication side effects, dietary changes, exercise recommendations, and potential specialist referrals can be incredibly helpful. When you arrive, you can preface the consultation with, "I've prepared a few questions to ensure we cover everything important for my management plan." Alternatively, some patients find it helpful to bring a trusted family member or friend to appointments. This person can act as a second set of ears, help to clarify points, and even prompt you to ask questions you might have forgotten. You could introduce this support by saying, "My [partner/friend/family member], [Name], is here with me today. They can help me understand the information and recall any important details." This introduces an additional advocate who can help ensure that the communication is clear and comprehensive.

When the core issue seems to be a lack of active listening, a gentle but direct approach to **highlight the need for their focused attention** can be beneficial. This involves making the provider aware that you perceive a disconnect without being accusatory. You might say, "I notice we've been discussing several important things, but I'm not sure we've fully addressed my concern about [specific issue]. Is it possible to spend a few more minutes on that?" or "I'm feeling a little concerned that my main issue might not have come across clearly. Could we take a moment to ensure we're on the same page regarding my [symptom/problem]?" This politely signals that you are not entirely satisfied with the current level of understanding. For example, if you've presented with a new, concerning symptom, and the provider has focused solely on prescribing a new medication for an existing condition, you might say, "I understand the new prescription for my [existing condition], but I'm still quite bothered by the new symptom of [new symptom]. I'm worried it could be related to [potential cause] and I'd like to discuss that further before we conclude." This directs the conversation back to the priority issue for you. In another scenario, imagine you've tried to explain a pattern of symptoms that seems to be worsening over time, and the provider's response has been to offer generic advice that doesn't seem to fit the progression you're experiencing. You could try saying, "I feel like the pattern of my symptoms has been evolving, and I'm not sure the current advice fully addresses how it's changed.

Can we review the timeline of my symptoms together so you can get a clearer picture?" By framing it as a desire to ensure they have the complete picture, you are inviting them to engage more deeply with the information you are providing.

If, after these attempts, you still feel your concerns are not being adequately addressed, it may be necessary to **request a different approach to explanation**. Sometimes, a provider's preferred method of communication, such as using highly technical jargon or providing very brief summaries, simply doesn't resonate with your learning style. Politely requesting a different way of understanding the information can make a significant difference. You could say, "I'm having a bit of trouble understanding the medical terms. Could you explain that using simpler language, or perhaps draw a diagram of what you mean?" or "Instead of a quick overview, could you walk me through the step-by-step process of what will happen during the procedure?" For instance, if a doctor is explaining the mechanism of a disease and is using complex biological pathways, you might ask, "Could you perhaps use an analogy to explain how this disease affects my body? I'm a visual learner and find analogies helpful." Or, if you are being given instructions for managing a complex treatment regimen, and the verbal explanation feels overwhelming, you might ask, "Would it be possible to get a written summary of the daily schedule for these medications and tests? That way, I can refer back to it easily." This not only helps you to grasp the information better but also shows the provider that you are committed to understanding and adhering to the plan, and that you require a different delivery method to achieve this.

In situations where communication breakdowns persist, it's also important to consider the provider's **non-verbal cues**. Sometimes, what a provider *isn't* saying or the way they are behaving can indicate a lack of engagement. Are they making eye contact? Are they rushing through your questions? Do they seem distracted or impatient? If you observe these cues, you might need to be more deliberate in your communication. You could try to gently interrupt a distraction by saying, "Excuse me, I see your phone is ringing, but I wanted to finish asking about..." or if they seem rushed, "I know you have a busy schedule, but this is important for my health. Could we take another five minutes to ensure I'm clear on this?" Acknowledging their busyness while still asserting the importance of your needs can sometimes prompt a shift in their focus. For example, if a provider is consistently looking at their computer screen while you are speaking, you might pause your explanation and then say, "I want to make sure I'm explaining this clearly, and I want to ensure you have all the information. Would it be helpful if I waited until you're looking this way?" This subtle redirect can bring their attention back to you. Another scenario might involve a provider who seems dismissive of your symptoms. You could try to counter this by providing objective data if possible. For instance, if you've been experiencing headaches and the doctor dismisses them as stress, but you've been meticulously tracking your blood pressure and have noted a correlation, you could say, "I understand you think it might be stress, but I've been tracking my blood pressure, and it seems to spike when the headaches are at their worst. Here are my readings for the past week." This evidence-based approach can sometimes prompt a more serious consideration of your reported symptoms.

Beyond your immediate concerns, it is also beneficial to **advocate for a clear understanding of next steps and follow-up**. Sometimes, communication breakdowns occur not during the discussion of the current issue, but in the lack of clarity about what happens next. If you leave an appointment feeling unsure about when to follow up, what symptoms warrant a call back, or what the next diagnostic or treatment milestone is, this itself is a communication gap. You should feel empowered to ask clarifying questions about this. For example, after discussing a new diagnosis, you could ask, "What are the specific signs or symptoms that would tell me I need to call the office before my next scheduled appointment?" or

"When should I expect to hear about the results of the tests we discussed today, and who will be contacting me?" This ensures that you have a clear roadmap for your ongoing care and know what to expect. Consider a situation where you've undergone a medical procedure. The post-operative instructions are crucial, but often patients are too groggy or overwhelmed to absorb them fully. Instead of simply nodding along, you might ask, "Could you please outline the specific signs of infection I should watch for in the first 48 hours, and what is the best way to contact you if I notice any of these?" This proactive approach to understanding follow-up care can prevent complications and ensure timely intervention if needed. Similarly, if a referral to a specialist has been made, clarifying the process is important: "Will the specialist's office contact me to schedule the appointment, or should I be reaching out to them, and if so, what information should I have ready?" This detailed approach to understanding the next steps ensures continuity of care and reduces the likelihood of important actions falling through the cracks.

Finally, cultivating a mindset where **seeking clarity is seen as a strength, not a weakness**, is fundamental. The healthcare system can sometimes feel hierarchical, making patients hesitant to question or challenge their providers. However, your role as the patient is to be an active participant in your own care. When you are clear about your health, your treatment, and what is expected of you, you are far more likely to achieve better outcomes. Therefore, if you find yourself in a situation where listening has fallen short, remember that it is your right and your responsibility to ensure you have the information you need. By employing strategies such as reiterating concerns, asking specific questions, using alternative communication methods, gently redirecting attention, and clarifying next steps, you are taking empowered action. These steps are not confrontational; they are communicative.

They are designed to bridge gaps, improve understanding, and ultimately foster a more collaborative and effective relationship with your healthcare providers. This proactive engagement transforms potentially frustrating encounters into opportunities for enhanced clarity and better health management, reinforcing the core principle of bidirectional listening.

4: Cultivating a True Patient-Provider Partnership

The journey of a patient-provider relationship often begins with a fundamental exchange of information. The patient presents with symptoms, concerns, and a history, while the provider offers expertise, comprehensive exam, diagnoses, and treatment plans. This transactional model, while necessary for the initial assessment and management of health issues, can sometimes limit the depth of engagement and the potential for optimal outcomes. However, the most effective patient-provider partnerships transcend this basic exchange, evolving into a dynamic arena of true collaboration. This shift from a mere information exchange to a collaborative endeavor which marks a significant maturation of the relationship, moving from a model where one party primarily imparts knowledge and the other primarily receives it, to one where both parties actively co-create the path forward for the patient's health.

This evolution into collaboration is not simply about politeness or improved bedside manner; it is rooted in the recognition that the patient is the ultimate expert on their own lived experience, their values, and their priorities. While the provider possesses invaluable medical knowledge and clinical experience, they do not live with the patient's condition day in and day out. They do not navigate the personal, social, and emotional complexities that accompany illness or the demands of a particular treatment regimen. Therefore, a truly collaborative approach acknowledges and leverages this unique patient expertise. It's about moving beyond the provider "telling" the patient what to do, to a process where both parties "decide together" what is best. This shared decision-making is the cornerstone of a collaborative partnership, where mutual respect for each other's knowledge and roles allows for the development of care plans that are not only medically sound but also personally meaningful and practically achievable for the patient.

Shared decision-making is characterized by a series of crucial interactions. First, the provider needs to present all reasonable medical options available for a particular condition or symptom. This isn't just about listing treatments; it involves clearly articulating the potential benefits, risks, side effects, and uncertainties associated with each option. For instance, when discussing management of type 2 diabetes, a provider might present lifestyle modifications (diet, exercise), oral medications (like metformin or sulfonylureas), and injectable therapies (like insulin or GLP-1 receptor agonists). Crucially, the provider must explain what each of these options entails – the dietary changes required, the frequency and potential side effects of medications, the commitment involved in regular exercise, or the learning curve for administering injections. Simply stating "you could take a pill or use insulin" is not sufficient. The patient needs to understand the nuances: "Taking metformin might cause some initial digestive upset, but it generally doesn't cause weight gain and has benefits for cardiovascular health. Insulin, on the other hand, requires regular blood sugar monitoring and injections, and carries a risk of hypoglycemia if doses aren't managed carefully, but it can be very effective in controlling blood sugar levels and preventing long-term complications."

Following the presentation of options, the provider must then actively elicit the patient's preferences and values. This is where the "shared" aspect truly comes into play. Questions like, "What are your main concerns about managing this condition?" "What are your priorities when it comes to your health right now?" or "How do you feel about taking daily medication versus making significant lifestyle changes?" are essential. For example, a patient might express a strong aversion to needles due to a phobia, or they might prioritize maintaining a certain level of physical activity over strict dietary adherence, or perhaps their work schedule makes it difficult to commit to a rigorous exercise routine. A patient with a busy, unpredictable travel schedule might find a daily pill easier to manage than an injection that requires refrigeration and specific administration times. Conversely, another patient might be highly motivated by quantifiable data and prefer to meticulously track their blood glucose levels and adjust insulin dosages, accordingly, finding a sense of control in this detailed management.

It's important to recognize that patient preferences are not static and can be influenced by a multitude of factors, including their understanding of the condition, their beliefs about health and illness, respecting religious beliefs, their social support system, their financial situation, their personal goals. A young parent might prioritize a treatment that allows them maximum energy to care for their children, even if it means more frequent appointments. An elderly individual living alone might prioritize a treatment that requires minimal self-management and has fewer potential side effects. A patient who is deeply concerned about the long-term impact of medications on their body might lean towards lifestyle changes, even if they are more challenging initially. Male patients need to understand which medications for blood pressure or mental issues will most likely affect their libido. The provider's role is to create a safe space for these preferences to be articulated and explored without judgment, facilitating a deep dive into what truly matters to the patient. This requires empathy and active listening, going beyond the surface-level responses to understand the underlying reasons for a patient's choices.

Once the options are understood and preferences are clarified, the next step is to reach a shared decision. This is a dialogue, not a dictation. The provider can offer their professional recommendation based on the clinical evidence and the patient's stated values, saying, "Given your preference for avoiding daily injections and your willingness to commit to dietary changes, I would recommend we start with [specific dietary plan] and [medication X]. My clinical experience suggests this combination has a high success rate for patients with your profile." However, the final decision rests with the patient, informed by this collaborative discussion. The provider can then support the patient in implementing the chosen plan, acknowledging that this is a joint undertaking. This process empowers the patient, fostering a sense of ownership over their health decisions, which in turn significantly boosts engagement and adherence to the treatment plan.

Given the plethora of information and new evolving technologies and treatments that are available no physician/ provider knows everything. If there is something new that a patient brings to you as a provider you have a right to gather ample research on the medication, product, device prior to giving a recommendation. I have no problem with telling a patient

I have never heard of that particular treatment. Where did you learn of it. I will tell my patient give me time to investigate the studies on the product or device and I will get back with you. My patients respect that answer and I give them a time frame that it may take me to get back with them with some type of answer. What the provider says is regarded as expert opinion so rather than just saying things or endorsing things without proper research on something you will do your patient who is relying upon you for solid answer a dis-service.

The benefits of this collaborative approach extend far beyond individual treatment adherence. Patients who feel actively involved in their care are more likely to trust their providers, feel respected, and experience greater satisfaction with their healthcare. This trust and satisfaction can lead to a more open communication channel, where patients feel comfortable sharing sensitive information or admitting when they are struggling with a treatment plan. This enhanced communication is crucial for identifying and addressing any emerging issues early, preventing potential complications or setbacks. For instance, if a patient has agreed to a new medication and is experiencing a subtle side effect that they initially dismissed as minor, a strong collaborative relationship built on trust and open dialogue encourages them to report it. The provider, in turn, can then adjust the treatment plan accordingly, reinforcing the patient's sense of agency and the partnership's effectiveness.

Moreover, collaborative decision-making can lead to more personalized and effective treatment plans. When a patient's lifestyle, preferences, and unique circumstances are integrated into the decision-making process, the resulting plan is more likely to be sustainable and successful. A plan that ignores a patient's work schedule, family responsibilities, or personal beliefs is often doomed to fail, not because it is medically flawed, but because it is practically unworkable for the individual. A collaborative approach ensures that the treatment plan is a good fit for the patient's life, increasing the likelihood of adherence and, consequently, better health outcomes. Imagine a patient with chronic pain who works a physically demanding job. A provider might initially suggest a medication regimen. However, through collaboration, the patient might reveal that the medication causes drowsiness, which is unsafe for their work.

The provider, understanding this critical piece of information, could then explore non-pharmacological approaches like physical therapy, or medications with different side-effect profiles, leading to a safer and more effective management strategy.

This shift towards collaboration also necessitates a re-evaluation of the provider's role. Instead of being the sole dispenser of medical authority, the provider becomes a facilitator, an educator, and a partner. They must be skilled in motivational interviewing, empathetic communication, and health literacy assessment. They need to be comfortable with uncertainty and the fact that the "best" decision may not always be the most obvious or the one with the highest statistical success rate, but rather the one that aligns with the patient's deeply held values and circumstances.

This requires a commitment to ongoing learning and adaptation, recognizing that each patient is unique and requires a tailored approach.

Furthermore, fostering collaboration means empowering patients to be active participants in their healthcare journey. This includes educating them about their conditions, explaining diagnostic processes, and making them aware of their rights and responsibilities within the healthcare system. When patients are well-informed, they are better equipped to engage in meaningful discussions with their providers, ask insightful questions, and advocate for their needs. This might involve providing patients with resources for further learning, such as reputable websites, patient advocacy groups, or educational materials. For example, after a diagnosis of heart disease, a provider might offer a patient a booklet on cardiac health, discuss a support group meeting, and explain the importance of understanding cholesterol levels and blood pressure readings, encouraging the patient to actively engage with this information.

The implementation of collaborative decision-making also requires addressing potential barriers. These can include time constraints in clinical practice, differing cultural beliefs, power imbalances inherent in the patient-provider dynamic, and a lack of training in communication and shared decision-making skills for healthcare professionals. Overcoming these barriers often involves systemic changes, such as increasing appointment times, integrating patient navigators, and providing ongoing professional development for providers. It also requires a cultural shift within healthcare organizations to prioritize patient-centered care and shared decision-making as core values.

Ultimately, moving from information exchange to collaboration transforms the healthcare experience. It shifts the focus from a disease-centric model to a patient-centric one, recognizing the individual's holistic needs. This partnership fosters a sense of shared responsibility and mutual respect, leading to increased patient satisfaction, improved adherence to treatment plans, and ultimately, better health outcomes. It cultivates a relationship where the patient is not a passive recipient of care, but an active, informed, and empowered partner in their own well-being, working hand-in-hand with their healthcare provider to achieve their health goals. This collaborative spirit is the bedrock upon which a truly effective and fulfilling patient-provider relationship is built, ensuring that care is not only effective but also deeply aligned with the individual's life and values.

At the heart of any thriving patient-provider partnership lies a deep wellspring of empathy and respect. These are not merely optional niceties; they are foundational pillars upon which trust is built, communication flourishes, and ultimately, healing is optimized. Moving beyond the purely clinical, this essence of human connection allows both parties to see beyond the diagnosis and the data, to the individual experiencing the journey of illness or wellness. Empathy, in this context, is the ability to understand and share the feelings of another. For the provider, it means actively striving to comprehend the patient's emotional landscape, their fears, their hopes, and the anxieties that often accompany health challenges. It's about recognizing that behind every symptom is a person grappling with a lived reality that is often far more complex than what can be gleaned from a medical chart.

Consider the patient facing a chronic illness diagnosis, perhaps diabetes or a debilitating autoimmune condition. While the provider might be adept at explaining the pathophysiology, prescribing medication, and outlining dietary recommendations, they may not fully grasp the day-to-day emotional toll. The patient might be experiencing feelings of grief for their former self, frustration with the limitations imposed by their condition, or a pervasive sense of uncertainty about the future. An empathetic provider will seek to understand these emotional undercurrents. This might manifest as actively listening when a patient expresses these feelings, validating their emotions with statements like, "It sounds incredibly difficult to be managing all of this," or "I can understand why you would feel worried about the long-term implications." It involves more than just acknowledging the patient's words; it's about attuning to the non-verbal cues—the hesitations, the downcast eyes, the subtle sighs—that can reveal a deeper emotional state. By demonstrating this understanding, the provider signals that the patient is seen not just as a collection of symptoms, but as a whole person whose emotional well-being is integral to their overall health.

Conversely, empathy from the patient's side is equally crucial. Patients often come into healthcare settings feeling vulnerable, perhaps even intimidated by the authority of medical professionals. They might have preconceived notions or past negative experiences that color their perception. An empathetic patient will make an effort to understand that their provider is likely managing a demanding schedule, dealing with numerous complex cases, and operating within the constraints of the healthcare system. This doesn't excuse poor communication or lack of attention, but it fosters a more charitable interpretation of any perceived shortcomings. An empathetic patient might recognize that a brief explanation is not necessarily a dismissal, but perhaps a need to move efficiently to the next patient or a consequence of limited appointment time. By approaching the interaction with an understanding of the provider's role and pressures, patients can communicate their needs more effectively and less confrontationally, paving the way for a more productive dialogue.

Respect forms the bedrock upon which empathy can truly flourish. It signifies acknowledging the inherent worth and dignity of each individual, regardless of their background, beliefs, or health status. For the healthcare provider, this means treating every patient with courtesy, dignity, and without judgment. It involves using respectful language, maintaining confidentiality, and ensuring that the patient feels heard and valued. This extends to respecting the patient's autonomy and their right to make informed decisions about their own bodies and health, even if those decisions differ from the provider's recommendations. For example, a patient might choose a less aggressive treatment option due to personal or philosophical reasons. A respectful provider will acknowledge this choice, explain its potential implications clearly, and support the patient in their decision without imposing their own views.

This could involve a dialogue like: "I understand you prefer to explore complementary therapies before starting medication. While the evidence for [specific complementary therapy] in treating your condition is still developing, let's discuss how we can monitor your progress closely and ensure we're addressing any worsening symptoms." This approach validates the patient's agency and fosters a sense of partnership rather than a hierarchical doctor-patient dynamic.

Respect also involves cultural humility and

awareness. Healthcare providers must recognize that patients come from diverse cultural backgrounds, each with its own unique beliefs about health, illness, healing, and death. What might be considered a standard or preferred treatment in one culture could be unacceptable or even offensive in another. For instance, some cultures may place a strong emphasis on traditional healing practices, while others may have specific views on end-of-life care or the disclosure of medical information. A provider who demonstrates cultural respect will inquire about these beliefs and integrate them into the care plan whenever possible. This could mean asking questions like, "Are there any traditional remedies or practices that you use that you'd like me to be aware of?" or "How do you and your family prefer to discuss sensitive health information?" By actively seeking to understand and accommodate these diverse perspectives, providers build bridges of trust and ensure that care is not only clinically effective but also culturally congruent and respectful.

From the patient's perspective, respect for the provider involves valuing their expertise and dedication. It means being punctual for appointments, providing accurate and complete information about one's health history, and engaging actively in the communication process. Respect also entails acknowledging the provider's professional boundaries and the demands of their role. For example, expecting immediate responses to non-urgent inquiries or dismissing the provider's advice without careful consideration can undermine the relationship. A respectful patient understands that the provider is a professional offering their best advice based on their training and experience. This doesn't mean unquestioning obedience, but rather a willingness to engage with the provider's guidance and to articulate any concerns or disagreements in a constructive manner.

The synergy between empathy and respect creates an environment where open and honest communication can thrive. When patients feel that their provider genuinely understands and cares about their situation (empathy) and treats them with dignity and consideration (respect), they are more likely to share crucial information, ask clarifying questions, and voice concerns that they might otherwise keep hidden. This can include admitting to not taking medications as prescribed, experiencing side effects, or feeling overwhelmed by a treatment plan. For example, a patient who feels respected might feel comfortable admitting, "I've been finding it really hard to stick to the new diet because my family doesn't eat the same way, and it feels isolating." An empathetic provider would respond not with judgment, but with understanding and problem-solving: "Thank you for sharing that with me. It's completely understandable that adjusting family meal dynamics can be challenging. Let's explore some strategies that might involve your family or provide you with more support to make this manageable."

Similarly, when providers demonstrate empathy and respect, patients feel empowered to be more active participants in their own care. They feel safe to express their preferences, values, and goals, which are essential for shared decision-making. This might involve a patient sharing that while a particular treatment is medically effective, it conflicts with their deeply held spiritual beliefs or lifestyle choices. An empathetic and respectful provider will not dismiss these concerns but will work collaboratively with the patient to find a solution that honors both the medical necessity and the patient's personal values. This collaborative spirit, born from empathy and respect, is what truly elevates the patient-provider relationship from a clinical transaction to a genuine partnership focused on the patient's holistic will-being.

The cultivation of empathy and respect is an ongoing process, requiring conscious effort from both sides of the healthcare encounter. For providers, it involves a commitment to active listening, non-verbal communication awareness, and cultural competency training. It means regularly reflecting on their own biases and assumptions and seeking to understand the patient's perspective as the primary source of information about their own experience. For patients, it involves approaching interactions with a mindset of openness, honesty, and a willingness to engage constructively with their healthcare team. By prioritizing these qualities, both patients and providers can build a stronger, more trusting, and ultimately more effective partnership that leads to better health outcomes and a more positive healthcare experience for all involved. This mutual understanding and regard are not just desirable; they are essential for navigating the complexities of health and illness together.

The transition from simply receiving medical advice to actively participating in health decisions is a significant shift, one that empowers patients and fosters a more robust patient-provider partnership. Shared decision-making (SDM) is not a passive reception of information; it is a dynamic, collaborative dialogue where both the patient and the healthcare provider bring their unique expertise to the table. The provider offers their clinical knowledge, understanding of medical evidence, and experience with various treatments. The patient, in turn, brings their intimate knowledge of their own body, their personal values, their lifestyle, their fears, their hopes, and their individual circumstances. When these two streams of expertise converge, truly informed and patient-centered decisions can be made.

Imagine a scenario where a patient, let's call her Sarah, is diagnosed with early-stage breast cancer. Her oncologist presents her with several treatment options, each with its own set of benefits and potential side effects. There's lumpectomy followed by radiation, mastectomy, and chemotherapy. For Sarah, this is an overwhelming deluge of information, presented in a language that is both technical and emotionally charged. This is where the practical application of shared decision-making becomes critical. The first step in this process, from the patient's perspective, is to feel comfortable and prepared to ask questions. It's about understanding that it is not only acceptable but encouraged to seek clarification.

For Sarah, this might mean asking her oncologist to explain each treatment option in simpler terms, avoiding jargon where possible. Instead of just hearing about "adjuvant chemotherapy," she might ask, "What exactly does chemotherapy do for my cancer, and what are the most common side effects I can expect to experience, both short-term and long-term?" This might involve inquiring about the success rates associated with each treatment option for someone with her specific cancer characteristics. She would also want to understand the implications of each choice on her daily life. For instance, "If I have a mastectomy, how will that affect my mobility and my ability to do physical activities I enjoy, like gardening or swimming?" or "What is the recovery time like for each of these surgeries, and what kind of support will I need during that period?"

Crucially, Sarah needs to understand how each option aligns with her personal values and her vision for her future. Perhaps she is a highly active individual who values her independence and wants to minimize any potential long-term impact on her physical capabilities. She might express this to her oncologist by saying, "My work involves a lot of physical activity, and I also love hiking and being outdoors. While I understand the need for effective treatment, I'm concerned about how these options might affect my ability to continue living an active life. What are the trade-offs in terms of long-term physical function for each of these choices?" Alternatively, her primary concern might be about the aesthetic impact of treatment, or the potential for recurrence, or the impact on fertility if she hopes to have children in the future.

The provider's role in this dynamic is to facilitate this exploration. They should not only present the medical facts but also actively inquire about the patient's priorities and concerns. This could involve using decision aids—tools specifically designed to help patients understand their options. These aids might include brochures, videos, or interactive websites that detail the benefits, risks, and uncertainties of each treatment. A skilled provider would guide Sarah through these resources, helping her to interpret the information and relate it back to her own situation. They would explicitly ask, "What are your main worries about treatment?" or "What are your goals for treatment, beyond just eradicating the cancer?" This might lead to a discussion about whether Sarah prioritizes minimizing the risk of recurrence at all costs, or if she is willing to accept a slightly higher risk in exchange for a better quality of life or less aggressive treatment.

Consider the process of weighing pros and cons. For Sarah, this isn't just a mental exercise; it's a structured conversation. The provider might offer a clear summary, perhaps even drawing a simple chart that outlines the key features of each option. For example, under "Lumpectomy + Radiation," the "Pros" might include "preserves breast appearance," "less invasive than mastectomy," and "high success rate." The "Cons" might list "requires daily radiation for several weeks," "risk of local recurrence," and "potential for radiation side effects like skin changes or fatigue." Similarly, for "Mastectomy," the "Pros" might be "removes more tissue, potentially reducing recurrence risk," and "avoids radiation side effects." The "Cons" could include "loss of breast, requiring reconstruction or prosthesis," "longer recovery time," and "potential for lymphedema."

Beyond these clinical factors, the conversation needs to delve into the less tangible aspects. What does “preserving breast appearance” mean to Sarah? Is it about vanity, or is it about her sense of self and body image? What does “quality of life” mean to her? Does it mean being pain-free, or being able to travel, or being able to work without significant fatigue? The provider needs to probe these subjective elements. They might ask, "If we go with the lumpectomy and radiation, how do you anticipate that impacting your daily routine? Would the daily trips to the radiation center be manageable for you, given your work schedule and family commitments?" Or, regarding mastectomy, "If you choose a mastectomy, how do you feel about the possibility of breast reconstruction? Is that something you would be interested in exploring, and what are your thoughts on that process?"

The decision-making process is rarely linear. Sarah

might initially lean towards one option, then have second thoughts as she considers new information or reflects more deeply on her priorities. It's important for her to feel that she can revisit her thoughts and that the provider is there to support her through this process, not to rush her into a choice. This might involve scheduling a follow-up appointment specifically to discuss her decision further, or offering a referral to a breast cancer support group where she can hear from other patients who have navigated similar choices.

The ultimate goal is for Sarah to arrive at a decision that she feels confident in, a decision that she believes is right for *her*. This sense of ownership over the decision is crucial for her adherence to treatment and her overall psychological well-being.

When patients feel they have genuinely participated in the decision-making process, they are more likely to follow through with the recommended plan, even when faced with challenges. They understand *why* they are doing what they are doing, and they feel their provider has respected their autonomy.

Another practical example can be seen in managing

a chronic condition like Type 2 diabetes. For a patient like John, who has recently been diagnosed, the provider might discuss lifestyle modifications versus medication. The provider could present the option of aggressive dietary changes and increased physical activity as a first-line approach, explaining the potential to manage blood sugar levels without medication. They would also present medication options, detailing their mechanisms of action, potential side effects (such as gastrointestinal upset or hypoglycemia), and their efficacy.

John's input is vital here. He might reveal that he struggles with consistency in his diet due to a demanding work schedule and frequent travel. He might say, "I love to cook, but when I'm on the road, it's hard to control what I eat. Fast food is often my only option, and I worry about that." He might also express his apprehension about taking daily medication, perhaps due to past negative experiences with medications or concerns about long-term side effects. He might ask, "Are there any natural or lifestyle approaches that have a strong track record for managing diabetes? I'd prefer to try those first if possible, before resorting to pills."

The provider's response would then be tailored to John's specific context. They might suggest resources to help him make healthier choices while traveling, such as apps that help locate healthier food options or tips for packing snacks. They might also explore specific types of diabetes medications that have fewer side effects or a simpler dosing schedule. Perhaps they would discuss metformin, explaining its mechanism, common side effects, and how it can be very effective in managing blood sugar. They might also introduce the concept of a continuous glucose monitor (CGM), which provides real-time data and can help John understand how his food choices and activity levels impact his blood sugar, making the lifestyle changes feel more concrete and rewarding.

The conversation could then move to weighing the pros and cons in a personalized way. For John, the "pro" of aggressive lifestyle changes might be avoiding medication, but the "con" is the significant effort required to change deeply ingrained habits and the potential for failure if he can't maintain consistency. The "pro" of medication might be greater certainty in blood sugar control, but the "con" is the potential for side effects and the need to remember to take it daily. The provider would help John articulate these trade-offs: "So, John, it sounds like your biggest concern with lifestyle changes is consistency while traveling, and with medication, it's the potential side effects and remembering to take it. How do you feel about trying a combination approach? We could focus on improving your diet as much as possible, and I could prescribe a medication that has a low risk of side effects and a simple dosing schedule, like once a day with dinner. We can then monitor your blood sugar closely and adjust as needed."

This collaborative approach allows John to feel that his concerns are being heard and addressed. He's not just being told to eat better; he's being offered practical solutions and a partnership in managing his condition. He can then make a choice that feels manageable and aligned with his capabilities and preferences. He might decide to try the combination approach, or he might feel confident enough to commit to a rigorous lifestyle change first, with the understanding that medication is an option if his efforts fall short. The key is that the choice is *his*, made with full awareness of the options and their implications.

Another area where shared decision-making is vital is in end-of-life care discussions. For a patient with a terminal illness, conversations about palliative care, hospice, or aggressive life-sustaining treatments are deeply personal and often emotionally charged. A provider would need to approach these discussions with immense sensitivity, ensuring that the patient's wishes and values are paramount. This might involve understanding what quality of life means to the patient, what their goals are for their remaining time, and what their fears are regarding pain, suffering, or loss of dignity.

A provider might initiate such a conversation by saying, "As we move forward, I want to make sure we are aligned with your goals for your care. What is most important to you at this stage of your illness? What are you hoping for in terms of comfort, pain management, and spending time with your loved ones?" This opens the door for the patient to express their preferences. They might state, "I don't want to be in pain, and I want to be able to talk to my family. I don't want any heroic measures if there's no chance of recovery."

The provider would then explain the available

options in relation to these expressed values. They could discuss palliative care services, which focus on symptom management and improving quality of life for patients with serious illnesses, and how that differs from hospice care, which is typically for patients with a prognosis of six months or less. They would explain the potential benefits and burdens of various medical interventions, such as artificial hydration, ventilation, or resuscitation, in the context of the patient's prognosis and stated wishes.

The decision-making process here is about ensuring that the patient's autonomy is respected until the very end. It might involve creating an advance directive or living will, a legal document that outlines the patient's wishes for medical treatment if they are unable to communicate them themselves. The provider's role is to ensure that the patient has all the necessary information to make these profound decisions, and to support them in communicating their choices to their family and their healthcare team. This requires not just medical expertise, but also a deep sense of empathy and a commitment to honoring the patient's wishes, even when they might differ from what the provider might personally choose.

The concept of "informed consent" is a cornerstone of shared decision-making, but it goes beyond a simple signature on a form. True informed consent means that the patient has been given sufficient information about the nature of the proposed treatment, the expected benefits, the potential risks and side effects, the alternative treatment options, and the likely consequences of not receiving any treatment. This information must be presented in a way that the patient can understand, and the patient must have the opportunity to ask questions and have them answered to their satisfaction. It also implies that the patient has the capacity to make such a decision and that their decision is voluntary, free from coercion or undue influence.

To facilitate this, providers should aim to make information accessible. This might involve using visual aids, providing written summaries, or recommending patient education materials from reputable sources. It also means being mindful of the patient's educational background, language proficiency, and cultural context. A patient who speaks limited English might require an interpreter, and a patient from a culture that views illness and treatment differently might need explanations that are culturally sensitive. For instance, in some cultures, it is customary for family members to be heavily involved in healthcare decisions, and a provider should be prepared to include them in the conversation if that is the patient's preference. Furthermore, shared decision-making acknowledges that medical knowledge is not always definitive. There are often uncertainties about the effectiveness of treatments, the likelihood of side effects, or the long-term prognosis.

Providers should be transparent about these uncertainties, explaining what is known, what is not known, and what the potential range of outcomes might be. This allows patients to make decisions that align with their tolerance for risk and their comfort level with uncertainty. For example, when discussing a new medication with limited long-term data, a provider might say, "While this medication has shown promising results in clinical trials, it's a newer treatment, and we don't have as much information about its effects over many years. We will monitor you very closely for any unexpected side effects." This honesty builds trust and allows the patient to participate in the decision with a realistic understanding of the unknowns.

The act of making a choice together also strengthens the patient-provider relationship. When patients feel heard, respected, and involved in their care, they are more likely to feel a sense of partnership. This can lead to greater adherence to treatment plans, better health outcomes, and increased patient satisfaction. It transforms the healthcare encounter from a transactional model, where the provider dispenses knowledge and the patient passively receives it, to a collaborative model, where both parties work together towards a common goal: the patient's health and well-being.

Practically, this can manifest in many ways. It means that at the end of a consultation, the provider doesn't just say, "Take this medication and come back in three months." Instead, they might say, "Based on our discussion and your preference for a treatment that minimizes travel, we've decided to try Medication X. The plan is to start with a low dose, and we'll check in next week by phone to see how you're doing with any potential side effects. Then, we'll schedule a follow-up appointment in a month to review your progress and make any necessary adjustments. How does that sound to you?" This approach confirms the shared decision and outlines a clear plan for ongoing care and communication.

It's also important to recognize that shared decision-making is an ongoing process, not a one-time event. As a patient's condition evolves, or as new information becomes available, treatment plans may need to be revisited and adjusted. The collaborative dialogue established through shared decision-making provides a strong foundation for these subsequent conversations, allowing patients and providers to adapt their strategies together as circumstances change. For example, if John's blood sugar levels are not adequately controlled with the initial combination approach, the provider would engage him again: "John, your recent blood tests show that your A1c is still a bit higher than we'd like. We have a couple of options: we could increase the dosage of your current medication, or we could consider adding a second medication that works differently. What are your thoughts on how to proceed?" This continues the partnership, ensuring that John remains an active participant in managing his diabetes.

Ultimately, cultivating shared decision-making is about empowering patients with the knowledge and the confidence to take an active role in their own health journey. It is a fundamental aspect of providing high-quality, patient-centered care, ensuring that medical decisions are not only clinically sound but also deeply aligned with the individual needs, values, and preferences of the person receiving care. By embracing this collaborative approach, both patients and providers can build stronger, more trusting relationships that lead to better health outcomes and a more fulfilling healthcare experience for everyone involved. It is the practical manifestation of a true patient-provider partnership, where every decision is made with shared understanding and mutual respect.

Building enduring alliances with your healthcare providers is a foundational element of proactive health management. Moving beyond the transactional interactions of seeking treatment, these long-term relationships cultivate a profound sense of continuity and personalized care. When your provider genuinely understands your medical history, your lifestyle, your family dynamics, and your personal values, they are better equipped to offer advice and interventions that are not just clinically sound, but also deeply resonant with your individual circumstances. This isn't about forming friendships, but rather about establishing a robust professional connection built on trust, respect, and consistent communication.

The cornerstone of any strong relationship is open and honest communication. For patients, this means proactively sharing updates about your health, even when you don't have a specific complaint. If you've tried a new diet, started a new exercise regimen, experienced a significant life event (like a stressful period at work or a family illness), or noticed subtle changes in your well-being, these are all pieces of information that can inform your provider's understanding of your overall health trajectory. Don't hesitate to bring these observations to your appointments. For instance, if you've been managing a chronic condition like hypertension and you've noticed that your sleep has been consistently disrupted due to stress, mentioning this to your doctor is crucial. They might not otherwise connect the dots between your sleep quality and its potential impact on your blood pressure management. Similarly, if you've adopted a new health-conscious habit, like incorporating meditation into your daily routine, sharing this can provide your provider with a more holistic view of your wellness efforts and allow them to offer encouragement or relevant advice, such as discussing how stress management can complement your existing treatment plan.

It's equally important to remain receptive to your provider's guidance and to follow through with agreed-upon treatment plans. When you consistently adhere to your prescribed medications, attend follow-up appointments, and implement lifestyle recommendations, you demonstrate a commitment to your health and a trust in your provider's judgment. This adherence allows your provider to accurately assess the effectiveness of treatments and make necessary adjustments. For example, if you are managing diabetes and consistently track your blood glucose levels and report them to your endocrinologist, they can see the impact of dietary changes or medication adjustments. This consistent feedback loop empowers them to fine-tune your treatment for optimal outcomes. Conversely, if you frequently miss appointments or deviate from treatment plans without discussing it with your provider, they may struggle to understand the root cause of any ongoing issues or make informed decisions about your care, potentially leading to suboptimal results or unnecessary complications.

Providing constructive feedback is another vital aspect of nurturing these professional bonds. Healthcare providers are human, and while they strive for excellence, there are always opportunities for improvement in how they communicate or manage patient care. If there was a specific aspect of your care that was particularly helpful, or if there's an area where you felt communication could have been clearer, sharing this feedback is invaluable. This could be done directly during an appointment, through a follow-up email, or via the clinic's patient feedback system. For instance, you might tell your primary care physician, "I really appreciated how you took the time to explain the different treatment options for my knee pain last month. Your diagram made it much easier to understand," or perhaps, "In our last appointment, I felt a bit rushed when discussing my medication side effects. Could we make sure to allocate more time for that discussion next time?" This type of feedback is not criticism; it's an investment in the continued quality of your care and an affirmation of your role as an active participant in your healthcare. It allows the provider to refine their approach and better serve you and other patients.

Building continuity of care means striving to maintain a consistent relationship with a primary care provider and, where possible, with specialists who are involved in your ongoing health management. While changing insurance plans or moving can sometimes necessitate a change in providers, making an effort to maintain these relationships whenever feasible yields significant benefits. A primary care physician who has known you for years understands your baseline health, your family history, your personal responses to various treatments, and any pre-existing conditions that might influence future health decisions. This deep understanding allows for more accurate diagnoses, more effective treatment planning, and a greater ability to identify subtle changes that might indicate emerging health issues.

Imagine a scenario where you develop a new symptom, like persistent fatigue. If you're seeing a new doctor who is unfamiliar with your history of hypothyroidism and your previous responses to levothyroxine dosage adjustments, they might explore a wider range of potential causes before considering the most likely one. However, a long-term provider would immediately consider your thyroid function as a primary suspect, leading to a faster and more accurate diagnosis.

Furthermore, this continuity extends to how information is shared. When you have a trusted provider, you are more likely to feel comfortable sharing sensitive personal information that might impact your health, such as details about your diet, exercise habits, stress levels, or even your social support system. This holistic information is crucial for effective care. For instance, if you are being treated for depression, admitting to your therapist that you've been experiencing significant financial strain and marital conflict provides essential context that can inform therapeutic strategies. A provider who knows your history is more likely to understand the nuances of your situation and offer tailored support, rather than a one-size-fits-all approach.

One practical way to foster this continuity is to be organized and prepared for your appointments. Keeping a running log of your medications, including dosage and frequency, any new supplements you're taking, and a summary of any significant health events or changes you've experienced since your last visit, can be immensely helpful. Bringing this information with you, perhaps in a notebook or a dedicated app on your smartphone, ensures that you don't forget anything important during the appointment. This preparation also allows your provider to have a comprehensive overview of your health status at a glance, maximizing the efficiency and effectiveness of your consultation time. For example, having a clear list of all your current prescriptions, including over-the-counter medications and supplements, can prevent potentially dangerous drug interactions that a busy physician might not recall from memory alone.

Remembering to ask questions is also a vital component of this ongoing relationship. Your provider is there to answer your concerns, and demonstrating that you are engaged and curious about your health encourages a more interactive and collaborative dynamic. Don't be afraid to ask for clarification if you don't understand something, whether it's a diagnosis, a treatment option, or a recommendation.

Questions like "Could you explain that in simpler terms?" or "What are the potential long-term effects of this medication?" or "What are the next steps in my treatment plan?" are all valid and important. Your provider should welcome these inquiries, as they signify that you are an active partner in your care.

When you consistently engage with your healthcare team, you build a rapport that transcends the clinical setting. This can lead to a deeper level of trust, where you feel more confident in their abilities and more comfortable sharing personal details that might otherwise remain private. This trust is essential, especially when navigating complex health issues or making difficult treatment decisions. For example, if you are considering a surgical procedure with significant risks, having a strong, trusting relationship with your surgeon can provide immense reassurance. You're more likely to believe their assessment of the risks and benefits and feel confident that they have your best interests at heart.

Another aspect of maintaining these relationships is being mindful of your provider's time and the clinic's policies. While your health is paramount, understanding that your provider also serves many other patients helps in managing expectations. If you have a minor query that can be addressed via a secure patient portal or a brief phone call, it might be more efficient than scheduling a full appointment. However, for anything that involves a new symptom, a change in treatment, or a complex discussion, a scheduled appointment is usually the most appropriate course of action. Respecting the healthcare system's structure ensures smoother operations and better care for everyone.

When it comes to specialists, maintaining continuity can be particularly challenging due to the often fragmented nature of specialty care. If you see multiple specialists, it's beneficial to have a primary care physician who can act as a central point of contact, coordinating care and ensuring that all your providers are aware of each other's interventions. You can also facilitate this coordination by requesting that copies of your specialist reports be sent to your primary care physician, or by bringing summaries of your specialist visits to your primary care appointments. This proactive approach helps to prevent any miscommunication or duplication of services. For instance, if you are seeing a cardiologist for a heart condition and an endocrinologist for diabetes, ensuring both are aware of any new cardiac medications prescribed by the cardiologist that could affect blood sugar control, or vice versa, is crucial.

In essence, building and maintaining long-term relationships with your care team is an ongoing process that requires active participation, open communication, and a commitment to continuity. It's about recognizing that your healthcare is not a series of isolated events, but rather a continuous journey. By investing in these relationships, you not only enhance the quality and personalization of your own care but also contribute to a more efficient and effective healthcare system. This consistent engagement ensures that your providers have the most comprehensive understanding of your health, enabling them to provide the best possible support and guidance throughout your life. It's a partnership where mutual understanding and shared goals pave the way for optimal health and well-being. This commitment to continuity also means being aware of the resources available to you. Many healthcare systems offer patient portals that allow you to access your medical records, communicate with your provider's office, request prescription refills, and even schedule appointments. Utilizing these tools effectively can significantly streamline communication and enhance your ability to stay connected with your care team. For instance, if you have a question about a lab result, you can often message your doctor directly through the portal and receive a response without needing to schedule a phone call or an in-person visit. This accessibility fosters a sense of constant connection and allows for timely intervention if necessary.

Furthermore, understanding the different roles within a healthcare team is also beneficial. Your primary care physician is your first point of contact for most health concerns and serves as the quarterback for your overall care. Specialists, on the other hand, have expertise in specific areas, such as cardiology, dermatology, or gastroenterology. Knowing when to consult a specialist, and ensuring that your primary care physician is involved in the referral process, helps to maintain a cohesive approach to your health. For example, if you develop a persistent rash, your primary care physician might be able to diagnose and treat common skin conditions. However, if the rash is unusual or doesn't respond to initial treatment, they would refer you to a dermatologist who can offer more specialized diagnostic and treatment options. Ensuring that the dermatologist communicates their findings and treatment plan back to your primary care physician closes the loop and provides your primary doctor with a complete picture of your health.

The transition of care is another critical juncture where long-term relationships prove their worth. Whether you are moving between healthcare facilities, being discharged from the hospital, or transitioning from pediatric to adult care, having a consistent provider who can help manage these transitions is invaluable. They can ensure that all necessary medical information is transferred accurately, that follow-up appointments are scheduled appropriately, and that you understand the new care plan. For example, when a patient is discharged from the hospital after surgery, their primary care physician can review the discharge summary, answer any questions the patient may have about post-operative care, and ensure that necessary follow-up appointments with surgeons or specialists are made. This smooth transition minimizes the risk of complications and ensures continuity of care.

In situations where multiple chronic conditions require management, the value of a long-term relationship with a primary care provider becomes even more pronounced. Managing conditions like diabetes, heart disease, and arthritis simultaneously can be complex, with potential interactions between different treatments and lifestyle recommendations. A provider who knows you well can help integrate the management of these conditions, ensuring that your overall treatment plan is cohesive and that interventions for one condition do not negatively impact another. For example, a patient with both diabetes and kidney disease might need specific adjustments to their blood pressure medications, as certain drugs effective for hypertension can be harmful to the kidneys. A primary care physician with a comprehensive understanding of the patient's history and the interplay between these conditions is best positioned to make these nuanced decisions.

Beyond the practical aspects of medical management, these enduring relationships also contribute to your emotional well-being. Knowing that you have a trusted healthcare professional who understands your concerns and respects your values can reduce anxiety and foster a sense of security. This is particularly true when facing serious or chronic illnesses. A provider who has been with you through various health challenges can offer not just medical expertise but also a sense of stability and reassurance. They become familiar with your coping mechanisms, your support system, and your personal resilience, allowing them to offer more empathetic and effective support. Imagine a patient undergoing chemotherapy for cancer. A relationship built on trust and open communication with their oncologist can make the difficult journey more bearable, as the patient feels understood and supported through the physical and emotional toll of treatment.

Finally, being an engaged and proactive patient is key to nurturing these relationships. This involves not only communicating openly and providing feedback but also taking responsibility for your own health by following through with appointments, adhering to treatment plans, and seeking information. When you demonstrate this commitment, you signal to your healthcare providers that you are a true partner in your care, fostering a dynamic that is mutually respectful and highly beneficial for your long-term health and well-being. This proactive stance empowers you to not only receive care but to actively shape it, ensuring that your healthcare journey is as effective, personalized, and positive as possible.

Navigating the complexities of the healthcare system, whether for oneself or for a loved one, can often feel like a daunting task. The sheer volume of information, the specialized terminology, and the inherent vulnerability that accompanies illness or injury can leave individuals feeling disempowered. However, cultivating a proactive stance and embracing the role of an advocate is not only possible but essential for securing optimal care.

This journey begins with understanding that you are an integral part of the healthcare team, and your voice, insights, and preferences matter profoundly.

One of the most critical aspects of self-advocacy and advocating for loved ones is the ability to communicate effectively and assertively. This doesn't imply aggression or confrontation, but rather a clear, respectful, and persistent articulation of needs, concerns, and preferences. When you are in a medical appointment, whether it's with a primary care physician, a specialist, or a nurse, remember that you have the right to be heard and understood. If a medical professional uses jargon you don't understand, don't hesitate to ask for clarification. Phrases like, "Could you explain that in simpler terms, please?" or "What does that medical term mean for my condition?" are perfectly acceptable and demonstrate your commitment to understanding your own health. Similarly, if a treatment plan is being discussed, and you have reservations or questions about its feasibility, potential side effects, or how it aligns with your personal values or lifestyle, it is your right to voice them. For instance, if a medication requires a complex dosing schedule that would be difficult to adhere to given your work commitments, or if a lifestyle change feels unsustainable, discussing these challenges openly with your provider can lead to a more realistic and effective plan.

This might involve exploring alternative medications with simpler regimens or discussing phased approaches to lifestyle modifications.

Empowering yourself also means understanding that seeking a second opinion is a standard and often advisable practice, especially when facing significant diagnoses or treatment decisions. It is not a reflection of distrust in your current provider but rather a prudent step to ensure you have explored all available options and have a comprehensive understanding of your condition. If you receive a diagnosis, such as a new cancer diagnosis or a recommendation for a major surgery, taking the time to consult with another specialist in the same field can provide valuable perspective.

This process can either reinforce the initial diagnosis and treatment plan, offering greater confidence, or it may reveal alternative approaches or additional considerations you hadn't previously encountered. When seeking a second opinion, be sure to bring all relevant medical records, including diagnostic test results, imaging reports, and the notes from your previous consultations. Clearly articulating your questions and concerns to the new specialist will facilitate a thorough and efficient evaluation. For example, if you were advised to undergo a specific surgical procedure, you might ask the second opinion physician, "Based on my current condition, what are the different surgical options available, and what are the potential outcomes and risks associated with each?"

Beyond immediate medical concerns, advocating for a loved one often involves navigating the complexities of their care when they may be unable to do so themselves, either due to cognitive impairment, severe illness, or other limitations. In such instances, having legal documentation like a Power of Attorney for Healthcare or an Advance Directive is crucial. These documents designate who has the authority to make medical decisions on behalf of the individual if they become incapacitated. Even without these formal documents, you can still be a vital advocate by actively participating in meetings, asking clarifying questions, and ensuring the care plan aligns with the person's wishes and values. For example, if your elderly parent is experiencing a decline in their health, you might attend their doctor's appointments and take notes, making sure to relay important information back to them and encouraging them to express their own preferences as much as possible. If a care facility is recommended, you would need to research facilities, ask detailed questions about staffing ratios, resident care plans, and emergency protocols, and advocate for an environment that meets their specific needs, whether that's related to dietary restrictions, mobility assistance, or social engagement.

Furthermore, becoming familiar with the healthcare system's infrastructure can significantly enhance your advocacy efforts. This includes understanding how to access your medical records, the process for filing grievances or complaints if necessary, and the services offered by patient advocacy departments within hospitals or healthcare organizations. Many hospitals have patient navigators or ombudsman services designed to help patients understand their rights, resolve issues, and navigate the system more effectively. If you feel that your concerns are not being adequately addressed, or if you encounter a situation where you believe standard protocols are not being followed, reaching out to these resources can provide valuable support and guidance. For instance, if you believe a medical error has occurred or if you are facing difficulties with billing and insurance that are impacting the continuation of care, a patient advocate can help mediate these issues and ensure your rights are protected.

The concept of "patient-centered care" is central to effective advocacy. This approach emphasizes treating patients as partners in their care, taking into account their individual needs, preferences, and values. When you are advocating for yourself or a loved one, you are essentially ensuring that this principle is upheld. This means not only discussing medical treatments but also considering the broader impact of illness on a person's life - their emotional well-being, their social support systems, their financial situation, and their spiritual beliefs. For example, if a patient with a chronic condition is struggling with the emotional toll of their illness, an advocate might ensure that mental health support services, such as counseling or support groups, are discussed and integrated into the care plan. Similarly, if a treatment requires significant lifestyle changes, an advocate might help explore how these changes can be realistically incorporated into the patient's daily life, perhaps by suggesting resources for nutritional counseling or accessible exercise programs.

Another crucial aspect of advocacy involves meticulously organizing and maintaining health information. This can include keeping a detailed record of all medical appointments, diagnoses, treatments, medications (including dosages and frequency), allergies, and test results. A well-organized binder or a secure digital health record can be invaluable, especially when dealing with multiple providers or during transitions of care, such as hospital admissions or discharges. When presenting this information to a new provider, it allows them to quickly gain a comprehensive understanding of your or your loved one's health history, minimizing the need for repetitive questioning and reducing the risk of missed information. For instance, having a clear list of all current medications, including over-the-counter drugs and supplements, is vital to prevent potential drug interactions. If your loved one is managing multiple chronic conditions, such as diabetes, heart disease, and arthritis, a centralized record can help all their providers understand how these conditions and their treatments might interact, leading to more coordinated and safer care.

When advocating for a loved one who has specific cultural or religious beliefs that influence their healthcare decisions, it is paramount to ensure these are respected and incorporated into the care plan. This might involve understanding dietary restrictions, preferences regarding modesty during examinations, or beliefs about end-of-life care. Openly discussing these aspects with the healthcare team from the outset can prevent misunderstandings and ensure that the care provided is sensitive and appropriate. For example, if a patient adheres to a strict kosher diet, an advocate would need to communicate this requirement to hospital nutrition services or the healthcare team managing their care to ensure compliant meal provisions. Similarly, if a patient has strong beliefs about the sanctity of life and wishes to avoid aggressive interventions, an advocate must clearly communicate these preferences to the medical team, particularly in critical care situations.

The role of an advocate also extends to questioning

the necessity and appropriateness of tests and treatments. While healthcare providers are trained professionals, it is always valid to ask, "Why is this test being recommended?" or "What are the benefits and risks of this particular treatment for me or my loved one?" This critical inquiry can help identify unnecessary procedures, prevent over-testing, and ensure that the most effective and least invasive options are considered first. For example, if a physician suggests a battery of tests for a seemingly minor symptom, an advocate might inquire about the diagnostic rationale for each test and whether a more focused approach could be taken initially. This proactive questioning can save time, reduce costs, and minimize patient exposure to potentially uncomfortable or risky procedures.

Moreover, understanding your insurance coverage and navigating the financial aspects of healthcare is an integral part of advocacy. This involves knowing what services are covered, what pre-authorization requirements exist, and what your out-of-pocket expenses might be. If you encounter issues with insurance claims, appeals processes, or unexpected bills, being prepared to communicate with the insurance company and, if necessary, with the healthcare provider's billing department is essential. Many patients find it beneficial to have someone assist them with these financial discussions, particularly if they are overwhelmed by medical bills or confused by insurance policies. For instance, if a particular medication or treatment is not covered by insurance, an advocate might work with the provider to identify alternative, covered options or explore patient assistance programs.

It is also vital to recognize that advocacy is not a one-time event but an ongoing process. As a person's health condition evolves, or as new treatments become available, the care plan may need to be revisited and adjusted. Maintaining open communication with healthcare providers and consistently reviewing and updating health information are key to ensuring that care remains aligned with the individual's needs and goals. This includes being prepared for follow-up appointments, actively participating in care plan reviews, and making sure that all members of the care team are informed of any significant changes in the patient's health or circumstances. For example, if a patient is transitioning from a hospital setting to home care, the advocate would ensure that the home health agency has all the necessary information from the hospital and that a clear plan for medication management, physical therapy, and follow-up medical appointments is established.

The power of documentation cannot be overstated in the role of an advocate. Keeping meticulous records of conversations with healthcare providers, including dates, times, names of individuals spoken to, and the substance of the discussion, can be incredibly helpful. This documentation serves as a factual record and can be crucial if any disputes or misunderstandings arise. It also helps in tracking progress and identifying patterns in care. For instance, if you are concerned about a recurring issue that seems to be inadequately addressed, having a record of previous discussions about the problem can support your case when you raise the concern again. This is particularly relevant when managing chronic conditions where subtle changes might occur over time that are easily overlooked without careful record-keeping.

Finally, advocating effectively requires a degree of

emotional resilience and self-care. The process can be stressful, demanding, and at times, emotionally draining.

Recognizing your own limits and seeking support when needed is not a sign of weakness but a strategic necessity. This might involve leaning on friends and family for emotional support, joining patient advocacy groups, or even seeking professional guidance for managing the emotional toll of caring for a loved one or managing your own health challenges. By prioritizing your own well-being, you are better equipped to be a strong and effective advocate for those who depend on you, ensuring that you can provide consistent and compassionate support throughout their healthcare journey. This proactive approach to self-advocacy and advocating for others transforms the patient-provider relationship into a true partnership, one where informed decision-making and personalized care are paramount.

5: Adherence, Outcomes, and Continuous Wellness

The intricate dance between a patient's commitment to a treatment plan and the ultimate success of that plan in achieving desired health outcomes is a fundamental principle in modern healthcare. This is not merely a matter of following instructions; it is a direct, causal relationship where consistent adherence acts as the linchpin for effective medical intervention. When individuals faithfully follow their prescribed medications, embrace recommended lifestyle modifications, and diligently attend scheduled follow-up appointments, they are actively participating in their own healing process. This proactive engagement is not simply about compliance; it is about empowering oneself to harness the full potential of medical advancements and therapies share with the patient by the expert in that subject matter. The impact of this dedication is profound, manifesting in tangible improvements in health, a reduction in the likelihood of complications, accelerated recovery times, and a significantly enhanced overall quality of life.

Many times, I have very frustrated patients come to

me after seeing their primary care physician or an urgent care provider about their ear, nose, and throat issue which has been going on for a few weeks to months. Their frustration is caused by the fact that they cannot tell me their diagnosis. I have to remind them that they are just supposed to answer the questions and give me the start of the problem, symptoms they are having, and any treatments they have tried. I reassure them they just have to let me know the above things and I will use my medical and procedural skills to discover what is going on with them. Patients in this new environment feel obligated to come with the problem, diagnosis, and treatment plan. That is not ideal medicine and can often times prolong the correct diagnosis and treatment plan.

Consider, for instance, the management of chronic conditions like diabetes. A patient diagnosed with Type 2 diabetes, for whom lifestyle changes and oral medication are prescribed, will experience vastly different outcomes based on their adherence. If this individual consistently monitors their blood glucose levels, adheres to a balanced diet, engages in regular physical activity as advised, and takes their prescribed medication on time, they are creating an environment conducive to stable blood sugar levels. This consistent management directly prevents the microvascular and macrovascular complications that plague uncontrolled diabetes, such as diabetic retinopathy, nephropathy, neuropathy, and cardiovascular disease. The absence of these complications preserves organ function, maintains vision, protects kidney health, and significantly reduces the risk of heart attack and stroke. In essence, adherence to the treatment plan acts as a shield, protecting the individual from the debilitating long-term consequences of the disease. Conversely, a patient who sporadically takes their medication, disregards dietary advice, or neglects exercise is far more likely to experience hyperglycemic crises, require more intensive interventions like insulin therapy, and ultimately develop the severe complications that can drastically reduce lifespan and quality of life. The direct link here is undeniable: adherence translates to better glycemic control, which in turn leads to the prevention of devastating complications.

The same principle applies across a spectrum of medical conditions. In the realm of cardiovascular health, for individuals prescribed antihypertensive medications to manage high blood pressure, consistent daily intake is critical. Blood pressure fluctuates throughout the day, and medications are designed to maintain a therapeutic level. Missing doses or taking them erratically can lead to periods of uncontrolled hypertension, increasing the risk of transient ischemic attacks (TIAs), strokes, myocardial infarctions, and heart failure. A patient who diligently takes their blood pressure medication as prescribed, alongside recommendations for reduced sodium intake and regular exercise, is actively working to keep their blood pressure within a healthy range, thereby safeguarding their cardiovascular system. This adherence not only prevents immediate crises but also contributes to long-term vascular health, reducing the cumulative damage that can occur from sustained elevated blood pressure. The outcome is a significantly lower risk of life-threatening cardiovascular events and a preserved ability to engage in daily activities without debilitating symptoms.

Furthermore, the impact of adherence extends to infectious diseases. For conditions requiring antibiotic treatment, such as bacterial pneumonia or urinary tract infections, completing the full course of prescribed antibiotics is paramount.

Antibiotics are designed to eliminate the bacteria causing the infection, but their effectiveness relies on maintaining a consistent concentration of the drug in the body over a specific period. If a patient stops taking their antibiotics as soon as they feel better, some bacteria may survive. These surviving bacteria can then develop resistance to the antibiotic. This phenomenon of antibiotic resistance is a growing global health crisis. A patient who adheres to their full antibiotic regimen is not only ensuring their own recovery but also contributing to the broader effort to combat antibiotic resistance. Non-adherence, on the other hand, can lead to treatment failure, a return of infection, the need for more potent and potentially toxic antibiotics, and the propagation of resistant strains of bacteria, making future infections harder to treat for everyone. This highlights how individual adherence has a direct impact on both personal health outcomes and public health.

The importance of adherence is also evident in the management of mental health conditions. For individuals managing depression, anxiety, bipolar disorder, or schizophrenia, consistent use of prescribed psychotropic medications is crucial for stabilizing mood, reducing psychotic symptoms, and improving overall functioning. These medications often require a period of weeks or months to reach their full therapeutic effect, and their withdrawal can lead to a rapid relapse of symptoms. A patient who consistently takes their antidepressant medication, attends regular psychotherapy sessions, and practices stress-management techniques is much more likely to maintain emotional stability, engage in social and occupational activities, and experience a higher quality of life. Conversely, sporadic medication use or discontinuation can result in a worsening of symptoms, increased risk of hospitalization, and a more challenging path to recovery. The direct link between consistent adherence to a multidisciplinary treatment plan and sustained mental well-being is a cornerstone of effective psychiatric care.

Beyond medications, adherence to lifestyle and behavioral recommendations plays an equally vital role in health outcomes. For individuals recovering from orthopedic surgery, for example, adherence to physical therapy protocols is critical. Following the prescribed exercises for range of motion, strengthening, and mobility not only facilitates proper healing of the surgical site but also helps prevent complications like stiffness, muscle atrophy, and deep vein thrombosis. A patient who diligently participates in their physical therapy sessions, performs home exercises as instructed, and gradually increases their activity levels will experience a faster and more complete recovery, regaining lost function and returning to their pre-operative activities sooner. Non-adherence, such as skipping therapy sessions or neglecting home exercises, can lead to prolonged recovery, persistent pain, joint stiffness, and potentially the need for further surgical intervention. The outcome is directly tied to the commitment to the rehabilitative process.

Similarly, adherence to dietary recommendations for conditions like kidney disease or inflammatory bowel disease (IBD) can profoundly influence disease progression and symptom management. Patients with chronic kidney disease are often advised to restrict their intake of potassium, phosphorus, sodium, and fluids. Strict adherence to these dietary guidelines helps slow the progression of kidney damage, reduce the accumulation of waste products in the blood, and manage fluid balance, thereby delaying or preventing the need for dialysis. For individuals with IBD, adherence to specific diets that avoid trigger foods, manage inflammation, and ensure adequate nutrition is essential for reducing symptom flare-ups, maintaining remission, and improving overall nutritional status and energy levels. The direct impact of these dietary choices on organ function, symptom severity, and quality of life underscores the critical role of patient engagement in managing complex chronic illnesses.

The importance of follow-up appointments cannot be overstated in this context. These appointments serve several vital functions: they allow healthcare providers to monitor the effectiveness of the treatment plan, assess for any adverse side effects, make necessary adjustments to medications or therapies, and provide ongoing education and support to the patient. A patient who consistently attends their follow-up appointments is ensuring that their care remains optimized and responsive to their changing health status. This proactive monitoring can catch potential problems early, before they become serious. For instance, in cancer treatment, regular follow-up appointments and diagnostic scans are crucial for detecting any recurrence of the disease or monitoring the side effects of chemotherapy or radiation. Adherence to this schedule provides early warning signs, allowing for timely intervention and potentially improving prognosis. Conversely, missing these appointments can lead to a delayed diagnosis of recurrence, unchecked progression of side effects, or a loss of therapeutic benefit from ongoing treatments. The outcome is directly influenced by the patient's commitment to the continuity of care.

The concept of "adherence" itself is multifaceted, encompassing not just taking medications but also adopting new behaviors, managing chronic conditions, and engaging in preventive health practices. For individuals with a history of cardiovascular disease, adherence to a heart-healthy lifestyle, including regular exercise, a diet low in saturated fats and cholesterol, and smoking cessation, is as crucial as taking prescribed medications. These lifestyle changes work synergistically with pharmacological interventions to reduce cardiovascular risk factors, improve endothelial function, and prevent future cardiac events. The patient who embraces these changes, despite the inherent challenges of habit formation, is directly contributing to their long-term cardiovascular health and reducing their susceptibility to heart attacks and strokes. This commitment to a healthier lifestyle, integrated with medical management, solidifies the link between adherence and positive health outcomes by fostering a holistic approach to well-being.

Furthermore, adherence is intrinsically linked to patient empowerment and self-efficacy. When patients understand the direct impact of their actions on their health outcomes, they are more likely to feel in control of their condition and motivated to adhere to their treatment plans. This understanding transforms them from passive recipients of care into active partners in their own health journey. For example, a patient with rheumatoid arthritis who understands how consistent adherence to disease-modifying antirheumatic drugs (DMARDs) and regular physical activity can prevent joint damage and preserve mobility is more likely to maintain these behaviors. The visible outcome of reduced inflammation, less pain, and preserved joint function reinforces the value of their commitment, creating a positive feedback loop that encourages continued adherence. This self-efficacy, fostered by understanding and witnessing the direct benefits, is a powerful driver of sustained adherence and, consequently, better health outcomes.

The complexity of modern medical regimens can sometimes present significant barriers to adherence. This is where the role of patient advocacy and effective communication with healthcare providers becomes critical. When patients or their advocates can openly discuss challenges with medication schedules, side effects, or the feasibility of lifestyle changes, healthcare teams can collaboratively develop more personalized and achievable plans. For instance, if a patient finds it difficult to remember to take multiple medications at different times of the day, a provider might suggest using a pill organizer, setting medication reminders on their phone, or exploring combination pills. If a recommended diet is proving too restrictive or unsustainable, a registered dietitian can be consulted to help create a modified plan that still meets nutritional needs. These adjustments, driven by open communication and a focus on adherence, directly improve the likelihood of successful outcomes by making the treatment plan more manageable and aligned with the patient's life.

In conclusion, the evidence overwhelmingly supports a direct and irrefutable link between patient adherence to treatment plans and positive health outcomes. From managing chronic diseases like diabetes and cardiovascular conditions to treating acute infections and mental health disorders, the consistent application of prescribed therapies, lifestyle modifications, and follow-up care is fundamental to achieving the best possible results. This adherence not only prevents complications, accelerates recovery, and enhances overall quality of life but also plays a crucial role in combating public health challenges such as antibiotic resistance. By fostering an understanding of this direct connection, empowering patients with knowledge and support, and encouraging open communication with healthcare providers, we can significantly improve the efficacy of medical interventions and promote a culture of continuous wellness. The patient, in their commitment to adherence, becomes an indispensable agent in their own health and recovery, directly shaping the trajectory of their well-being.

The journey toward optimal health and sustained wellness is rarely a straight path. While the science behind medical treatments and lifestyle interventions is robust, the human element - the patient's ability and willingness to adhere to these recommendations - introduces a layer of complexity. Recognizing and addressing the myriad barriers that can impede adherence is therefore not just a matter of good practice, but a critical component of ensuring that medical interventions achieve their intended positive outcomes. Without acknowledging these obstacles, even the most scientifically sound treatment plan is destined for suboptimal results.

One of the most significant and pervasive barriers to adherence is the financial burden associated with healthcare. Prescription medications, specialist consultations, diagnostic tests, and recommended medical equipment can accumulate a substantial cost, even for individuals with insurance. For those without adequate coverage or with high deductibles and co-pays, the decision to adhere to a treatment plan can become a daily calculus of necessity versus affordability. For instance, a patient prescribed a life-saving medication for a chronic condition like heart failure may find the monthly cost prohibitive. If they must choose between paying for the medication and covering other essential living expenses like rent or groceries, adherence is inevitably compromised. This economic strain can lead to patients rationing their medication, skipping doses, or altogether discontinuing treatment, directly jeopardizing their health and increasing the likelihood of costly hospitalizations or emergency interventions down the line. Similarly, the cost of specialized dietary foods, physical therapy equipment, or even reliable transportation to appointments can erect insurmountable financial walls, effectively barring individuals from fully participating in their own care.

Beyond the direct financial costs, the complexity of treatment regimens themselves can be a formidable obstacle. Modern medicine often involves multiple medications, each with different dosing schedules, specific instructions for administration (e.g., with or without food), and potential interactions with other drugs or substances. A patient managing several chronic conditions, such as diabetes, hypertension, and hyperlipidemia, might be prescribed half a dozen different pills, each to be taken at distinct times of the day. Navigating this pharmaceutical maze requires a high degree of organization, memory, and understanding. For individuals with cognitive impairments, learning disabilities, or simply a demanding daily schedule, remembering to take each medication correctly can be an overwhelming task. This complexity can lead to inadvertent errors, such as missed doses, double-dosing, or taking medications at the wrong time, all of which can reduce efficacy or increase the risk of adverse events. The sheer number of pills, combined with instructions like "take with food," "take on an empty stomach," or "avoid dairy," can create a cognitive load that makes consistent adherence a significant challenge.

The physical and psychological toll of medication side effects also plays a crucial role in adherence. While medications are designed to treat illness, they can also produce a range of unwanted effects, from mild gastrointestinal upset and fatigue to more severe reactions like dizziness, tremors, or mood changes. Even seemingly minor side effects, if persistent or particularly bothersome, can significantly impact a patient's quality of life and motivation to continue taking the medication. For example, an antidepressant that causes persistent drowsiness might make it difficult for a patient to work or engage in daily activities. Similarly, a pain reliever that leads to constipation or nausea can make the prospect of taking it each day unappealing.

When side effects outweigh the perceived benefits, or when they interfere with a patient's daily functioning, discontinuing the medication becomes a logical, albeit often detrimental, choice. The fear of experiencing these side effects can also be a preemptive barrier, leading some individuals to avoid starting or continuing a prescribed treatment even before experiencing any issues.

A lack of understanding regarding the condition, the treatment plan, or the rationale behind specific recommendations is another significant impediment to adherence. If a patient does not grasp why a particular medication is necessary, how it works, or what the long-term consequences of non-adherence might be, they are less likely to be motivated to follow through. This can stem from inadequate patient education, language barriers, or simply a lack of engagement from the healthcare provider.

For instance, a patient with a urinary tract infection who is prescribed a course of antibiotics but isn't fully informed about the importance of completing the entire course may stop taking the medication as soon as their symptoms subside, believing they are cured. This incomplete treatment can lead to a recurrence of the infection and, more critically, can contribute to the development of antibiotic-resistant bacteria, a growing public health crisis. Similarly, a patient advised to modify their diet to manage a chronic illness might not understand the specific links between certain foods and their symptoms or the long-term health implications of dietary choices.

Furthermore, various psychosocial factors can create significant hurdles. Social isolation, lack of a strong support system, and stressful life events can all undermine a patient's ability to prioritize and manage their health. For individuals living alone or those with limited social connections, the practical and emotional support needed to adhere to complex regimens might be absent. A patient who has recently experienced a job loss, a divorce, or the death of a loved one may find their focus shifting away from managing their chronic condition, leading to a decline in adherence. These life stressors can create a cascade effect, making it harder to maintain healthy routines, remember medications, or attend appointments. Inequities in access to care, often stemming from socioeconomic status, geographic location, or cultural background, also contribute to adherence challenges. Individuals in rural areas, for example, may face long travel distances to reach healthcare facilities or pharmacies, making regular visits and prescription refills difficult.

The inertia of established habits and the challenge of behavior change cannot be underestimated. Our daily lives are governed by routines, and adopting new behaviors, such as regular exercise, dietary changes, or meticulous medication schedules, often requires significant effort to break old patterns and establish new ones. For someone accustomed to a sedentary lifestyle, starting an exercise program can feel daunting and inconvenient. Similarly, someone who enjoys sugary snacks might struggle to adhere to a diabetic-friendly diet. These ingrained habits represent a powerful force that can resist even the most well-intentioned efforts at change. The perceived inconvenience or difficulty associated with these changes can lead to procrastination and eventual abandonment of the new behaviors, even when the long-term health benefits are clear.

Recognizing these diverse barriers is the first crucial step. The subsequent, and arguably more critical, step is to equip patients and healthcare providers with practical strategies and coping mechanisms to navigate and overcome these obstacles. A fundamental strategy for enhancing adherence is the promotion of open and honest communication between patients and their healthcare providers. Patients must feel empowered to voice their difficulties without fear of judgment. This includes discussing financial concerns, side effect experiences, challenges with understanding instructions, or any other personal obstacles they are facing. For instance, if a patient expresses that the cost of their medication is too high, a pharmacist or physician can explore alternative, more affordable generic options, discuss patient assistance programs, or investigate if a different, less expensive medication with similar efficacy exists. This collaborative approach ensures that the treatment plan is not only medically sound but also practically achievable for the individual.

To address the complexity of medication regimens, various practical tools and techniques can be employed. Pill organizers, often with compartments for each day of the week and specific times of day, can significantly simplify medication management. Setting timed alarms or reminders on smartphones or using dedicated medication reminder apps can serve as consistent prompts. For patients with limited technological access or literacy, simple visual cues, such as placing the pill bottle next to their toothbrush or breakfast plate, can be effective. Healthcare providers can also consolidate medication schedules where possible, prescribing combination pills or suggesting times that align with the patient's existing daily routines, such as taking a blood pressure pill with their morning coffee. The pharmacist's role in patient education, providing clear instructions and answering questions at the point of dispensing, is also invaluable in demystifying complex medication schedules.

When side effects become a barrier, the key is often proactive management and adjustment. Instead of discontinuing a medication altogether, patients should be encouraged to report any adverse effects to their healthcare provider promptly. The provider can then assess the severity of the side effect and consider several options. This might include adjusting the dosage, switching to a different medication within the same class that has a different side effect profile, or prescribing an additional medication to manage the side effect itself (e.g., an anti-nausea medication for a chemotherapy patient). For side effects that are temporary, such as initial fatigue from an antidepressant, providing reassurance and a timeline for improvement can help patients persist. Education about what to expect can also mitigate anxiety and improve tolerance.

Improving understanding is a continuous process that requires tailored educational approaches. Healthcare providers should utilize plain language, avoiding medical jargon, and confirm comprehension by asking patients to rephrase information in their own words. Visual aids, such as diagrams of how a drug works, videos demonstrating proper inhaler technique, or written materials in the patient's preferred language, can greatly enhance learning.

For patients with literacy challenges, verbal explanations and hands-on demonstrations are crucial. It's also beneficial to involve family members or caregivers in the education process, as they can provide support and reinforcement at home. Regularly checking in with patients about their understanding and addressing any misconceptions that arise during follow-up visits is equally important.

Addressing psychosocial barriers often requires a more holistic approach that extends beyond the clinical encounter. Healthcare providers can screen for social determinants of health, such as housing instability, food insecurity, or lack of social support, and connect patients with appropriate community resources, social workers, or patient navigators. Encouraging patients to build or engage with their support networks, whether through family, friends, or patient support groups, can provide both emotional and practical assistance. For individuals experiencing significant life stressors, mental health support or counseling may be necessary to help them cope and maintain focus on their health. Recognizing that adherence is influenced by a patient's overall life circumstances allows for more empathetic and effective interventions.

Overcoming the inertia of habits and facilitating behavior change involves a focus on gradual, achievable steps and building self-efficacy. Instead of demanding a complete overhaul of lifestyle, providers can encourage incremental changes. For example, for a patient aiming to increase physical activity, starting with a goal of a 15-minute walk three times a week is far more attainable than aiming for an hour at the gym daily. For dietary changes, suggesting the addition of one healthy meal or eliminating one unhealthy beverage per day can be more manageable than a complete dietary overhaul. Motivational interviewing techniques, where the healthcare provider guides the patient to explore their own reasons for change and identify solutions, can be highly effective. Reinforcing successes, no matter how small, and celebrating milestones can build confidence and sustain motivation. The development of a personalized action plan, collaboratively created by the patient and provider, that outlines specific, measurable, achievable, relevant, and time-bound (SMART) goals, can provide a clear roadmap for change.

Furthermore, leveraging technology and community resources can offer innovative solutions to adherence challenges. Telehealth appointments can reduce travel burdens and make it easier for patients to access specialist care or follow-up consultations. Mobile health (mHealth) applications can provide reminders, track progress, offer educational content, and even facilitate communication with healthcare teams. Community pharmacies can play a vital role by offering medication management services, counseling, and acting as accessible touchpoints for patients. Local support groups and non-profit organizations dedicated to specific chronic conditions can offer invaluable peer support, shared experiences, and practical advice, fostering a sense of community and shared purpose.

Finally, it is crucial to acknowledge that adherence is not a static state but a dynamic process that may fluctuate over time. Patients may face periods of high adherence followed by challenges due to new life events, changes in their condition, or shifts in their motivation. Therefore, ongoing assessment and reinforcement are essential. Regular follow-up appointments provide opportunities to re-evaluate adherence, identify emerging barriers, and adjust strategies as needed. A supportive and non-judgmental approach from healthcare providers, coupled with patient engagement in problem-solving, can create a positive cycle that fosters sustained adherence and ultimately leads to improved health outcomes and a better quality of life. By proactively addressing these barriers with empathy, creativity, and a commitment to patient-centered care, healthcare systems can significantly enhance the effectiveness of treatments and empower individuals to achieve their wellness goals.

The therapeutic relationship, at its core, is built on a foundation of trust and mutual respect. When patients feel that their healthcare providers genuinely care about their well-being and are invested in their journey toward recovery or better health management, a powerful catalyst for adherence is ignited. Positive interactions are not merely pleasantries; they are potent therapeutic tools that can transform a patient's perspective on their treatment plan, fostering a sense of partnership rather than a passive reception of directives. Imagine a scenario where a patient, hesitant and anxious about a new diagnosis, is met with a physician who listens attentively, validates their concerns, and explains the treatment in a clear, reassuring manner.

This initial encounter sets a tone that can profoundly influence the patient's subsequent engagement with their care. The physician's empathy, their willingness to answer questions thoroughly, and their clear articulation of the benefits and expectations of the treatment can demystify the process and empower the patient to move forward with confidence.

This sense of empowerment is a cornerstone of adherence. When patients feel heard and understood, they are more likely to internalize the recommendations given to them. A simple act, like a nurse taking the time to explain the purpose of a medication beyond just its name and dosage - perhaps detailing how it works to alleviate specific symptoms or prevent future complications - can create a deeper understanding and appreciation for the treatment's value. This deeper understanding moves adherence from a chore to a conscious, informed decision. Consider the impact of a pharmacist who not only dispenses medication but also engages the patient in a brief, encouraging conversation about managing side effects or integrating the medication into their daily routine. Such interactions, however brief, can reinforce the patient's commitment and provide them with practical, actionable advice that makes adherence feel less daunting.

Moreover, positive reinforcement from healthcare professionals plays a critical role in maintaining motivation. When a patient achieves a milestone, however small – perhaps successfully managing a chronic condition for a month, or adhering to a new exercise regimen without interruption – a word of encouragement from their doctor or a congratulatory note from a nurse can be incredibly affirming. This positive feedback loop validates their efforts and strengthens their resolve to continue. It's akin to a coach cheering on an athlete; the external validation fuels internal motivation. This is particularly crucial for chronic conditions where adherence is a lifelong commitment. Patients need to feel that their ongoing efforts are recognized and valued, not just their initial engagement with the treatment plan.

The emotional climate of a healthcare setting also contributes significantly to a patient's willingness to adhere. A warm, welcoming atmosphere, coupled with staff who exhibit patience and kindness, can reduce patient anxiety and foster a more positive outlook on their treatment. Conversely, a hurried, impersonal, or dismissive interaction can leave a patient feeling devalued and discouraged, making them less likely to engage fully with their care. For instance, a patient attending regular physical therapy sessions might find their motivation waning due to the sheer effort required. However, if their therapist consistently greets them with enthusiasm, celebrates their progress, and creates a supportive environment where they feel safe to express their challenges, the patient is far more likely to continue attending and to push themselves to achieve better results. The therapist's positive demeanor can transform a potentially arduous experience into one that is empowering and rewarding.

This emphasis on positive interactions extends to all members of the healthcare team, from receptionists who greet patients with a smile to the specialists who conduct complex procedures. Each touchpoint contributes to the overall patient experience and, by extension, their adherence behavior. A patient who feels treated with dignity and respect at every stage of their healthcare journey is more likely to trust the advice and recommendations they receive. This trust is paramount. When trust is established, patients are more open to discussing sensitive issues, admitting to non-adherence, and collaborating with their providers to find solutions. This open dialogue is essential for adjusting treatment plans, managing side effects effectively, and ultimately achieving optimal health outcomes.

Consider the impact of shared decision-making, a concept intrinsically linked to positive interactions. When healthcare providers involve patients in the decision-making process, asking for their preferences, values, and goals, and then jointly developing a treatment plan, adherence rates often improve. This approach acknowledges the patient as an active participant in their own health, rather than a passive recipient of care. For example, when discussing lifestyle modifications for diabetes management, a provider who asks about the patient's cultural food preferences and work schedule, and then tailors the dietary and exercise recommendations accordingly, is more likely to see sustained adherence than a provider who imposes a generic, one-size-fits-all plan. This collaborative spirit fosters a sense of ownership over the treatment plan, making patients more invested in its success.

The nuances of communication are also critical. Beyond just conveying information, the way that information is delivered can significantly impact its reception.

Empathetic listening, where providers reflect back what they've heard to ensure understanding and validate the patient's feelings, can create a powerful connection. Phrases like, "I understand that you're feeling overwhelmed by the number of medications you need to take," or "It sounds like the side effects are really impacting your daily life," can open the door for more honest conversations and problem-solving. This type of communication builds rapport and demonstrates that the provider sees the patient as a whole person, not just a collection of symptoms or a diagnosis.

Furthermore, healthcare professionals can actively cultivate an environment of optimism and hope, which are powerful motivators for adherence. When patients are facing serious illnesses or challenging treatment regimens, a provider's hopeful yet realistic outlook can be instrumental. Sharing success stories of other patients who have navigated similar challenges, or focusing on the potential benefits and improvements in quality of life that the treatment can bring, can instill a sense of possibility. This is not about false promises, but about highlighting the efficacy of the treatments and the patient's own capacity to overcome obstacles with the right support.

The role of the entire healthcare team in creating these positive interactions cannot be overstated. A coordinated effort where all members understand the importance of patient engagement and possess the necessary communication skills ensures a consistent and supportive experience. This includes training healthcare professionals in communication techniques such as motivational interviewing, active listening, and patient-centered care. When these skills are integrated into daily practice, they foster an environment where patients feel empowered, respected, and motivated to actively participate in their health and wellness journey. Ultimately, positive interactions are not just a "nice to have" in healthcare; they are a fundamental component of effective treatment, driving adherence, improving outcomes, and enhancing the overall patient experience.

5.1 Monitoring Progress and Adjusting the Plan

The journey toward optimal health and sustained wellness is rarely a linear path. It's more akin to navigating a dynamic landscape, where terrain can shift, requiring constant awareness and the willingness to adapt. Once a treatment plan is established, the crucial work of monitoring progress and making necessary adjustments begins. This isn't a passive waiting game; it's an active, ongoing collaboration between you and your healthcare team. Understanding how to effectively track your own progress, recognize signs that a plan may need modification, and communicate these observations is paramount to achieving and maintaining your health goals.

The first step in this continuous process is establishing clear metrics for success. What does improvement look like for you? This can vary dramatically depending on your specific health condition, the goals of your treatment, and your individual circumstances. For someone managing chronic pain, progress might be measured by a reduction in the intensity or frequency of pain episodes, an improved ability to perform daily activities, or a greater sense of control over their condition. For an individual focused on weight management, progress could be tracked through weight loss, a decrease in specific body measurements, improved cholesterol levels, or increased energy. For a patient managing a mental health condition, indicators might include a reduction in the frequency or severity of depressive or anxious episodes, improved sleep patterns, better concentration, or a greater capacity to engage in social activities.

It's vital to work with your healthcare provider to define these measurable outcomes. These should be realistic, achievable, and aligned with your personal values and lifestyle. Simply stating a goal like "feel better" is too vague for effective monitoring. Instead, try to quantify it. For instance, if you're aiming to improve sleep, a measurable goal might be to fall asleep within 30 minutes of going to bed at least five nights a week, or to experience no more than one nighttime awakening per night. For cardiovascular health, a provider might set a target blood pressure range or a specific cholesterol level that needs to be achieved. These concrete benchmarks provide a clear target and a tangible way to assess whether the current plan is delivering the desired results.

To facilitate this monitoring, keeping a health journal or log can be an incredibly powerful tool. This doesn't need to be an exhaustive daily record of every sensation, but rather a focused documentation of key information relevant to your treatment. What to include in your log will depend on your condition and treatment plan. For some, it might involve tracking medication intake, noting any side effects experienced, and recording their severity and duration. For others, it might be about logging physical activity, dietary intake, blood glucose levels, mood, or specific symptoms. The act of writing things down not only creates a valuable record for your provider but also enhances your own awareness of your body's responses and patterns. For example, a patient with migraines might log the date, time, duration, intensity, potential triggers (food, stress, sleep patterns), and the effectiveness of any treatments used. Over time, this journal can reveal subtle connections and patterns that might otherwise go unnoticed, providing crucial insights for treatment adjustments.

When tracking physical symptoms, be as objective as possible. Instead of writing "felt bad," describe the symptoms in detail: "experienced a sharp, stabbing pain in my left knee for 2 hours, rated 7 out of 10 in intensity, which limited my ability to walk." Similarly, if you are monitoring your mental state, instead of "felt sad," try to articulate specific feelings or behaviors: "felt a pervasive sense of hopelessness, had difficulty concentrating at work, and lacked the energy to engage in hobbies for three consecutive days." The more precise your observations, the more valuable they will be to your healthcare team.

It's also important to monitor not just the presence or absence of symptoms, but also your functional capacity and overall quality of life. Is the treatment plan enabling you to do more of the things you enjoy or need to do? Are you experiencing more good days than bad days? Are you feeling more engaged and present in your life? These subjective measures, while harder to quantify, are often the most meaningful indicators of a successful treatment plan. For someone recovering from a serious illness, progress might mean being able to walk to the mailbox without becoming excessively fatigued, or being able to participate in a family gathering for an extended period. These are vital aspects of wellness that should not be overlooked.

Regular follow-up appointments with your healthcare provider are the lynchpin of effective progress monitoring. These appointments are not just for dispensing prescriptions; they are structured opportunities to review your progress, discuss any challenges, and make informed decisions about the next steps. Come prepared for these appointments by bringing your health log or notes. Be ready to openly and honestly discuss what you've observed. Don't hesitate to share both positive developments and any setbacks or concerns. It's common for treatment plans to require fine-tuning. What works perfectly at the outset might become less effective over time, or new challenges might emerge that were not initially anticipated.

Recognizing when a plan needs adjustment is a

critical skill. Several indicators might suggest that your current treatment approach isn't optimal. If your symptoms are not improving as expected, or if they are worsening despite consistent adherence to the plan, this is a clear signal that a change may be needed. For example, if a medication prescribed to lower blood pressure is not achieving the target range, or if an exercise program designed to improve stamina isn't yielding the desired results, these are indications that the dosage, type of medication, or nature of the exercise might need to be revised.

Similarly, if you are experiencing new or unmanageable side effects that are significantly impacting your quality of life, this warrants a discussion with your provider. While some side effects are expected and can often be managed, severe or persistent ones can be a sign that the current medication or treatment modality isn't the best fit. For instance, if a medication causes debilitating nausea, dizziness, or a rash that interferes with daily activities, it's important to inform your doctor. They may be able to adjust the dosage, switch to a different medication with a potentially better side-effect profile, or explore alternative treatment options.

Another sign that an adjustment might be necessary is a plateau in progress. You might have experienced initial improvements, but then reached a point where you are no longer seeing any further gains. This can happen in many health conditions, from weight loss to rehabilitation after an injury. It doesn't necessarily mean the plan has failed, but rather that the body may have adapted, and a new stimulus or approach is required to break through the plateau. Your healthcare provider can help identify if this is the case and suggest modifications, such as increasing the intensity of exercise, altering dietary patterns, or introducing a new therapeutic technique.

Furthermore, changes in your life circumstances can also necessitate a review of your treatment plan. New stressors, significant life events (like a change in job, a loss of a loved one, or a new relationship), or the development of other health conditions can all influence how you respond to your current treatment. For instance, increased stress levels can exacerbate symptoms for many chronic conditions, from irritable bowel syndrome to anxiety disorders. In such situations, the existing treatment plan might need to be supplemented with stress management techniques or adjustments to medication dosages.

Your provider will play a crucial role in guiding these adjustments. They will consider your progress data, your reported experiences, and their clinical expertise to determine the best course of action. This might involve:

Modifying Medication: This could mean adjusting the dosage (increasing or decreasing), changing the frequency of administration, or switching to an entirely different medication within the same class or a different class altogether. For example, if an antidepressant is not providing sufficient relief, the dose might be increased, or a different type of antidepressant might be tried.

Altering Lifestyle Recommendations: If the current diet or exercise plan isn't yielding results or is proving unsustainable, modifications will be made. This could involve changing the types of foods recommended, adjusting calorie intake, modifying exercise routines to include different activities or intensity levels, or incorporating new behavioral strategies.

Introducing New Therapies or Interventions: Sometimes, the current plan might need to be augmented with additional therapies. This could include physical therapy, occupational therapy, psychotherapy, complementary therapies like acupuncture or massage, or the use of assistive devices.

Setting New Goals: As you achieve initial health objectives, new goals may be set to continue progressing toward optimal wellness. For example, once a certain weight loss target is met, the focus might shift to maintaining that weight, building muscle mass, or improving cardiovascular fitness.

It is essential to maintain open and honest communication with your healthcare team throughout this process. Don't be afraid to voice your concerns or ask questions about the rationale behind any proposed changes. Understanding *why* a particular adjustment is being recommended can increase your confidence in the plan and improve your adherence. For example, if your doctor suggests a higher dose of a medication, ask them to explain the expected benefits and any potential increased risks associated with the higher dose. Similarly, if a new exercise is recommended, ask about how it complements your existing routine and what specific benefits it is intended to provide.

The collaborative nature of healthcare means that you are an active partner in making these decisions. Your insights into your own body and how you feel are invaluable.

While your provider offers medical expertise, you are the expert on your own experience. Therefore, sharing your observations, your adherence challenges, and your personal goals is crucial for developing a treatment plan that is not only medically sound but also practical and sustainable for your life.

Embracing the dynamic nature of health management is key. Health is not a static state, and your treatment plan should be viewed as a living document that evolves as you do. Regular monitoring, honest communication, and a willingness to make adjustments are fundamental to navigating your wellness journey effectively. By actively participating in this process, you empower yourself to take control of your health, optimize your treatment, and achieve lasting well-being. This proactive approach ensures that your care remains tailored to your needs, maximizing the chances of success and helping you to live your healthiest, most fulfilling life. The continuous feedback loop between your experience and your provider's expertise creates a powerful synergy, driving progress and adapting to the ever-changing landscape of your health.

The journey toward optimal health, as we've explored throughout this book, is not a destination but a continuous voyage. It's a lifelong commitment to your well-being, a dynamic process of learning, adapting, and actively engaging with your health. This isn't about achieving a perfect state of being that remains unchanged, but rather about cultivating a robust and resilient approach to life that embraces the inevitable ebb and flow of health. Empowered wellness means recognizing that you are the primary architect of your health, equipped with the knowledge and agency to make informed decisions and to steer your course with purpose. It's about transforming from a passive recipient of care into an active partner, one who understands their condition, their treatment, and their own vital role in achieving and maintaining a high quality of life.

This active participation is rooted in a proactive mindset. It means not waiting for a crisis to engage with your health, but rather integrating healthy habits and mindful awareness into your daily existence. This proactive stance involves consistently applying the strategies we've discussed: diligent adherence to treatment plans, meticulous monitoring of progress, and open, honest communication with your healthcare team. It's about building a robust foundation of self-care that can withstand the challenges that life inevitably throws your way. Think of it as tending to a garden; regular watering, weeding, and attention to the soil are far more effective than waiting until the plants are wilting to intervene. Similarly, consistent engagement with your health, even when you feel well, is crucial for preventing setbacks and fostering long-term vitality. This proactive approach also extends to seeking out new information, staying abreast of advancements in your specific condition or general wellness, and continually refining your understanding of what supports your individual needs.

A cornerstone of this empowered approach is the cultivation of a strong patient-provider partnership. The insights you gain from tracking your symptoms, understanding your medications, and recognizing your body's signals are invaluable. When you bring this self-knowledge to your appointments, you transform the interaction from a simple check-in to a collaborative strategy session. Your healthcare providers are experts in their fields, offering critical medical knowledge and experience. However, you are the undisputed expert on your own lived experience, your unique physiology, and your personal response to treatments. This duality of expertise is what creates a truly effective partnership. By sharing your observations, your challenges with adherence, and your personal goals and values, you enable your provider to tailor your care with unprecedented precision. They can then offer not just a medically sound plan, but one that is also practical, sustainable, and aligned with your life circumstances and aspirations. This collaborative dialogue ensures that the treatment plan remains a living document, one that is continuously refined to meet your evolving needs and to maximize its effectiveness.

Embracing this journey also means fostering a mindset of resilience and adaptability. There will be days when adherence feels effortless, and days when it feels like a monumental task. There will be periods of significant progress, and periods where progress seems to stall. These fluctuations are normal, and they are not indicators of failure. Instead, they are opportunities to learn and to adjust. When you encounter a hurdle, instead of becoming discouraged, view it as a chance to reassess your strategies. Perhaps a particular adherence technique isn't working for you anymore, or a new stressor has entered your life that is impacting your energy levels. This is the time to engage in self-reflection, consult your health journal, and reach out to your healthcare provider to discuss potential modifications. The ability to bounce back from setbacks, to learn from them, and to adjust your approach is a hallmark of empowered wellness. It's about developing the mental fortitude to persist, even when the path becomes challenging.

Continuous learning is another vital component of this lifelong journey. Our understanding of health and medicine is constantly evolving. Staying informed about new research, treatment options, and best practices relevant to your health condition is essential. This doesn't mean becoming your own doctor, but rather becoming an informed consumer of healthcare information. It involves critically evaluating sources, discussing new information with your provider, and being open to exploring evidence-based advancements that could improve your outcomes. For example, if you manage a chronic condition like diabetes, staying updated on new insulin delivery systems, continuous glucose monitoring technology, or dietary research can significantly enhance your management strategies. Similarly, for mental health, understanding advancements in psychotherapeutic techniques or the nuances of different medication classes can empower you to have more informed conversations with your therapist or psychiatrist. This commitment to continuous learning ensures that your approach to wellness remains current and optimized.

Furthermore, empowered wellness extends beyond the clinical setting to encompass the broader aspects of your life that influence your health. This includes your social connections, your environment, your financial well-being, and your overall sense of purpose and meaning. Nurturing strong relationships, creating a supportive living space, managing financial stress, and engaging in activities that bring you joy and fulfillment all contribute significantly to your health. These elements can often feel like separate domains, but in reality, they are deeply intertwined with your physical and mental well-being. For instance, social isolation can exacerbate symptoms of depression and anxiety, while a supportive community can provide encouragement and practical assistance. Similarly, living in an environment with access to healthy food options and safe places to exercise can significantly impact your ability to adhere to healthy lifestyle choices. Recognizing these interconnectedness and taking steps to optimize these broader life factors is an integral part of a holistic, empowered wellness approach.

The practice of mindfulness and self-compassion plays a crucial role in sustaining this lifelong journey. Being mindful means paying attention to your thoughts, feelings, and bodily sensations without judgment. This practice can help you to better understand your internal cues, recognize early signs of stress or illness, and respond to your needs more effectively. It also allows you to observe your own adherence patterns and internal dialogue without harsh self-criticism. Self-compassion involves treating yourself with the same kindness, understanding, and acceptance that you would offer to a dear friend facing similar challenges. It acknowledges that setbacks are a part of the human experience and encourages you to be gentle with yourself during difficult times. This can be particularly important when managing chronic conditions, where the demands of self-care can be significant. Cultivating self-compassion can prevent burnout and foster a more sustainable and positive relationship with your health journey. It allows you to acknowledge the effort you are putting in and to forgive yourself when you fall short of your own expectations.

The ultimate goal of empowered wellness is not just the absence of disease, but the presence of vitality, resilience, and a high quality of life. It's about living fully, engaging meaningfully with the world, and experiencing a sense of well-being that permeates all aspects of your existence. This is achieved by consistently applying the principles of proactive self-care, informed decision-making, and collaborative partnership with your healthcare team. It's about recognizing that your health is an ongoing project, one that requires your sustained attention, your evolving knowledge, and your unwavering commitment. As you continue on your path, remember that you are not alone. Your healthcare providers are your allies, and the knowledge you have gained from this book is a powerful tool in your arsenal. By embracing your role as an empowered participant, you unlock the potential for a healthier, more fulfilling, and more vibrant life, not just today, but for all the years to come. This continuous engagement ensures that your wellness journey remains a source of strength and fulfillment, enabling you to navigate life's complexities with confidence and grace, and to truly thrive.

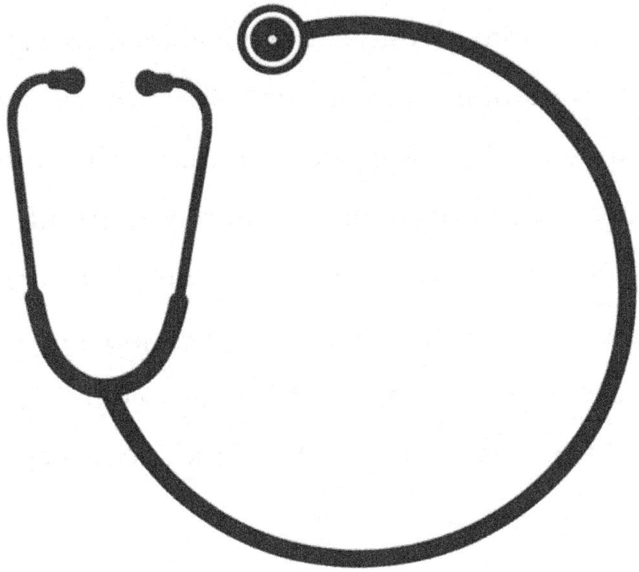

Glossary

This glossary defines key terms and concepts introduced throughout the book, providing clear and concise explanations to enhance your understanding of empowered health management.

Adherence: The extent to which a person's behavior matches agreed-upon recommendations from a healthcare provider.

Empowered Wellness: An active, informed, and participatory approach to managing one's health, characterized by agency, self-advocacy, and collaboration with healthcare providers.

Mindfulness: A mental state achieved by focusing one's awareness on the present moment, while calmly acknowledging and accepting one's feelings, thoughts, and bodily sensations.

Patient-Provider Partnership: A collaborative relationship between a patient and their healthcare provider, built on mutual respect, shared decision-making, and open communication.

Proactive Health Management: Taking initiative to prevent illness and promote well-being through consistent healthy habits and informed engagement with healthcare, rather than reacting to existing conditions.

Resilience: The capacity to recover quickly from difficulties; toughness. In a health context, it refers to the ability to adapt and bounce back from challenges, setbacks, or illness.

Self-Advocacy: The act of representing one's own interests and needs, particularly in healthcare settings.

Self-Compassion: The ability to be kind, understanding, and accepting of oneself, especially during times of suffering or perceived failure.

References

The information presented in this book is supported by a robust foundation of scientific research and clinical guidelines. The following are key references that informed its content, offering avenues for deeper exploration and verification of the principles discussed.

World Health Organization. (2023). Patient Empowerment. https://www.who.int/patient-empowerment

Institute for Healthcare Improvement. (2022). The Science of Improvement. https://www.ihi.org/resources/Pages/AboutIHI/ScienceofImprovement.aspx

Sapolsky, R. M. (2017). Behave: The Biology of Humans at Our Best and Worst. Penguin Books.

Kabat-Zinn, J. (2013). Full Catastrophe Living: Using the Wisdom of Your Body and Mind to Face Stress, Pain, and Illness. Bantam Books.

Langer, E. J. (2005). The Power of Mindful Learning. Harvard University Press.

Christensen, C. M., Bohmer, R. M., S Kenagy, J. W. (2000). Will doing more healthcare for you really result in better health? Harvard Business Review, 78(5), 142-151.

About the Author

Charla V. Johnson is a seasoned, licensed, and certified Physician Assistant healthcare professional and patient advocate with over 24 years of experience dedicated to improving patient outcomes and fostering a more collaborative healthcare landscape especially in underserved communities and minorities. Holding a master's in business administration degree in healthcare, and master's degree in theology along with a bachelor's degree in physician assistant science.

Charla V. Johnson has worked across various healthcare settings, from clinical practice in military medicine, to private practice, to major healthcare systems. Driven by a passion for patient empowerment, she has focused on translating complex medical information into accessible strategies that enable individuals to take an active role in their health journey. She has established a successful medical podcast on YouTube @bodynbalance25 and on TikTok @25bodynbalance where she shares valuable health information for patients. Her motto is ***"I tell you things your doctor doesn't have time for in the office!"***

Through extensive research, direct patient

interaction, and a commitment to evidence-based practices, Ms. Johnson has developed a deep understanding of the challenges and triumphs inherent in managing personal well-being. This book represents a distillation of that knowledge, aiming to equip readers with the tools and confidence to become true partners in their own healthcare.

When not engaged in advocacy or writing, Ms. Johnson enjoys working with her local and national church, e.g., spending time with family, enjoying basketball games, walks on the beach, and researching for her weekly podcast.

Made in the USA
Monee, IL
06 April 2026

47815705R00167